A Practical Treatise

of

Astral Medicine

and

Therapeutics

M. Duz, M.D., D.A.

Fellow of the N.A.S. of the U.S.,
and Honorary Member of the
Homeopathic Institute of Bogota, Columbia

First published: 1912
Current edition: 2014

ISBN-10: 0-86690-652-5
ISBN-13: 978-0-86690-652-4

Cover Design: Jack Cipolla

Published by:
American Federation of Astrologers, Inc.
6535 S. Rural Road
Tempe, AZ 85283

www.astrologers.com

Printed in the United States of America

Dedication

To the National Astrological Society of the U.S.A.,
this book is affectionately dedicated.

General Disclaimer

This book is provided for information purposes only, with no guarantee of accuracy; it is not intended as a substitute for medical advice, nor as a claim for its effectiveness in treating any symptoms or disease. If symptoms persist, seek professional medical advice; minor symptoms can often be a sign of a more serious underlying condition. Homeopathic remedies are very dilute, and while the homeopathic remedy may be beneficial, the raw product may be harmful.

Herbal and homeopathic substances can be harmful if taken in excess or with other medication. Some substances used in herbal and other remedies are poisons that can lead to death if taken in the wrong dosage. Others can cause severe illness if taken inappropriately. A little knowledge can be dangerous.

AFA does not accept any responsibility for the consequences of any action taken as a result of any of the content of this book, and makes no warranties regarding the value or utility of the information and resources contained in this book.

Contents

Preface

The science of the stars, which is a law of Nature, has for its aim the establishing of the relations existing between terrestrial phenomena and stellar configurations, which Shakespeare calls the planets' *mixture*. These relations are those of probability, so that being fixed on such or such combination of heavenly bodies we are right to attain the production or manifestation of such or such physical and psychical phenomena, present or future, because in nature all links together, all fastens, all reproduces.

This is the object of my present labour, where I will collect all that may be useful in a practical way. I do not think that a cultivated spirit, free from prejudiced ideas, may not subscribe to a science which deals with the causes for judging of the effects. The causes necessarily hold of the sidereal phenomena on which depend those of the terrestrial things, and when we study the former we study the latter.

M. Flambart, of the Polytechnic College of France, considering the laws governing heredity and atavism from the astrological standpoint, arrives at a result which is amazing; on the other hand, the Rev. B. Hicks, of St. Louis, establishes on the same basis his long range weather and earthquake forecasts which are proving most accurate.

The great difficulty for us was nevertheless to obviate, for a practical science like medicine, the tedious calculations and the personal interpretations that astrology is heir to. These complications would have discouraged the most willing physicians and particularly the non-medical public.

After many researches, I thought that the best way was that of mere experience, as the astral tradition concerning medicine is unfortunately lost in the night of past ages, albeit the Hippocratic as well as the ancient Egyptian teachings are founded upon it.

As to the humoural principle I have adopted, I will say, not being blemished of archaism, that far from being in opposition to the modern scientific data, it is a simpler and comprehensible expression of them. In fact, we do not regard the diseases otherwise than the ancients when we ascribe to them an origin: an intoxication, an infection, the presence of toxins, of ptomains, of leucomaines, etc., which perfectly correspond with the different qualities invested by the humours (peccant humours). The only difference existing between them and ourselves is that they generalize when we particularize.

And Dr. Perrier, of Lyons, in his thesis on astrological medicine, says: "Undoubtedly the spirits have been darkened by the most foolish superstitions, but it would be inadmissible that the general consensus was coarsely deluded during so many centuries. It was said that error is never universal."

The author is especially indebted to the learned editor of *Old Moore's Monthly Messenger* and to the distinguished treasurer of the National Astrological Society of the U.S.A., Dr. Walter H. Lewis of Manchester New Hampshire, for their encouragements and expressions of interest in the realization of his arduous task, for which he addresses here his feelings of gratitude and thankfulness.

Chapter I

Generalities

There are more things in heaven and earth, Horatio.
Than are dreamt of in your philosophy.—Shakespeare

The object of the astral medicine is to establish the medical practice on fixed data, controllable at will, and to get at the causes of things often escaping observation, but apparent in their effects. Hence our error. Thus the railway passenger sees running away hedges, trees, fields, when none of these objects move from their places. But this optical illusion does not prevent him from reaching the termination of his voyage, as do those who reason through the effects in making progress through the sciences. Nevertheless, the defect of this manner or reasoning by interverting the parts is to damage the principles and conclusions, which, not being in accordance with the reality, strain the reason and lead into erroneous judgments.

Going up to the primary causes, the science of the stars reveals the true meaning of the facts, and so does the astral medicine in regard to the medical practice.

Thus, in *physiology* it gets out the role of the cell and that of the humours; in *pathology*, it opens new horizons as to the individual constitution and its genesis, and synthesizes the nosological scale; in *hygiene*, it indicates the true way to be followed; in *climatology*, it betrays the favourable or unfavourable conditions and periods of seasons and days, etc.; in *therapeutics*, it furnishes a law in harmony with nature, that of similars; and last but not least, in *sociology*, it gets out the natal dispositions of our children and serves to guide their tendencies in social life. Now in support of the well-founded basis of this science, which is far from being a delusive one, I may cite a few of the most eminent ancient and modern authorities who duly considered, patronized, and practiced it. These authorities are: Thales, Anaximander, Pythagoras, Hippocrates, Democritus, Anaxagoras, Eudoxus, Ptolemy, Galen, Avenzoar, Averroes. Artephius, Arnold of Villanova, Paracelsus, Canlan, Lord Bacon, Tycho-Brahe, Kepler, and the most celebrated French chemist, Chevreul, who, in his analysis of Artephius' *Key of the Mighty Wisdom*, says: "The predominating idea in him is the indifference of the matter to affect such or such a propriety. Being one, it must owe the qualities it revests under certain circumstances to various influences coming from outside causes. And this idea directly leads to the admission in fact, of the transmutation of all sublunary bodies in each other, and subsequently to the acknowledgment of the astral influences upon them." And he adds: "There is no alchemical work which may be compared to *The Key of the Mighty Wisdom* as to the intensity of the speculative view with its application to the transmutation and the astral influences upon the sublunary bodies."

The elements of the ancients are four: water, air, fire, and earth, to which they assignated the qualities: cold, moist, hot, or dry. Their elements correspond to ours, which are in the same order: hydrogen, nitrogen, oxygen, and carbon, and their qualities synthetise the four essential and fundamental operations of Nature, which respectively are:

1. Congelation
2. Volatisation
3. Combustion
4. Condensation

2

These result from the combination of the elements in various degrees.

All then in nature brings back to these elements to which hydrogen and carbon serve as radicals. And however hidden be life in its principle, it is obvious that it is not less intimately fastened, through immediate and necessary links, to most of the agents of the outward world--water, air, fire, and earth--and to the forces animating them--heat, light, electricity, and magnetism. These latter put it in correlation with the Universe, confirming thus Hermes' aphorism: "What is below is like that which is above, and what is above is like that which is below, for the accomplishment of the same thing."

Just as for all beings and earthly things, at his conception, man is stamped with the qualities, properties, pathological states and vices suitable to the medium and the elements which surrounded him at his birth environment. "Man is born," says Fioravanti, "under his element, and in the course of his life is dominated by it."

This is what forms his constitution, which is unalterable, while his temperament is variable and modifiable according to the age, the physical and moral education, the medium where he is living, the alimentation, the training, etc.

There is the reason that each nation, each country, each collectivity, has its own temperament; because all individuals subdued to the same regimen and environment are identically modelled and bear a similar stamp. Notwithstanding, in reality, each one will betray his own temperament, although it would be grafted on that of the masses.

The temperament, as well as the constitution, depend on the blood and its manner of being. In fact, it does not suffice through exercise, training, or diet, to develop an organ or splanchnic cavity to the cost of another organ or cavity for contending to have in the same time modified the individual temperament, i.e., as to render a thoracic one, an abdominal, etc. The temperament cannot be modified but through time, when the blood and its qualities are modified. That is the reason why it often denotes the constitution.

The temperaments are four in number, and they are:
1. The lymphatic; quality, cold
2. The sanguine; quality, moist
3. The bilious; quality, hot
4. The nervous and melancholic; quality, dry

Nevertheless, the nervous and melancholic temperament, being but an exaggeration of the bilious, can be reduced to three, thus corresponding to the following classification:
1. Temperament of insufficient nutrition (apathetic, feeble people)
2. Temperament of equilibrated exchanges (active, energetic, healthy people)
3. Temperament of incomplete elimination (sensitive, nervous, cositive people)

Still, the quaternary division is to be preferred as suiting better to the practical purposes.

They are the abdominal organs which prevail in the lymphatic temperament; hence, circulatory slowness, lesser caloric, and slackness of the fibres of the thoracic organs (lungs, heart), although they are pretty well developed.

The thoracic organs (lungs, heart) are predominating in the sanguine temperament; hence, more energetic circulation and igneous fluid.

With the bilious, the liver and its functions are brisk; hence, more energetic circulation and stronger caloric than with the sanguine.

The nervous and melancholic temperament has the cranium or brain more developed than the abdominal and thoracic organs, which are contracted; hence, circulatory difficulty and lesser caloric, through portal and splenic trouble and diaphragmatic and hypochondriac spasm.

Often, the inspection of the face betrays the temperament. So the forehead responds to the brain; the mouth, the chin, and the lower part of the cheeks to the abdomen; and the eyes, the nose, and the upper part of the cheeks to the thorax.

Yet these organismic unfoldings appoint the temperament and not the constitution. Surely this latter holds equally of an organismic origin, as does the temperament. But while this latter depends on the organic volume, the former is heir to the cell, and the qualities it gets through the sidereal influences having presided at the birth.

Hence, seven constitutions, which are:
1. The encephalic, depending on the nervous system (nervous influx)
2. The cardiac
3. The thoracic
4. The cranio-abdominal, or stomachic, depending on the solar plexus, called the abdominal brain
5. The hepatic
6. The splenic
7. The renal

And as the constitution is but the diathesis constituting the organismic, hereditary, or atavic drawback, so these seven divisions are as well diathesic.

The diseases in their beginning are submitted to the same elements concurring to the formation of the constitutions, and invest their character and nature. Then each one evolves on the individual constitution; so the measles, for instance, of Peter, typically differs from that of Paul, and requires a different treatment, although the nosological entity is the same in both. Hence the aphorism: "There are no diseases, but diseased." (Hahnemann. Peter)

Besides, for the existence of a morbid state, it is indispensable that the cellular equilibrium be troubled.

The organs or principal centres presiding over the physiological functions are:
1. The abdominal organs
2. The thoracic organs
3. The thoraco-abdominal organs
4. The cephalic organs

There is the natural evolutional order of diseases which primarily generated in the abdominal organs (first step), attain afterwards the circulatory organs and the sanguification (second step), and then produce a want of oxydation in tissues (third step), troubling the nervous influx-innervation (fourth step) which is the result of a humoural conflagration, and so the more complex one of the nosological scale.

The therapeutics which comprehend the hygienic measures and the pharmaceutical agents withstanding the morbid manifestations, proceed of the same principles ruling the constitutions and diseases, and pull all the same their efficacy in curing ailments of the sidereal influences, as they assume the elementary qualities of the heavenly bodies presiding over each one. Consequently, the medicines call on seven groups, which are:
1. The Solar group
2. The Lunar group
3. The Mercury group
4. The Venus group
5. The Mars group
6. The Jupiter group
7. The Saturn group

"The remedy," says Hippocrates, "entered in the body, operates on the humour which is most analogous to its nature; it afterwards attacks the others and purges them."

Two therapeutical laws govern the medicine and are fundamental. The first is that of contraries: "*Contraria Contrariis curantur*"; and the second that of the similars: "*Similia Similibus curantur.*"

Yet neither the contrary nor the similar of a thing exist in nature, although the hot opposes the cold, and the moist the dry. So brought to the elementary qualities of beings and things, these laws acquire a practical meaning and sense. In fact, the pain due to an inflammation and the inflammation itself, may heal through cold or hot applications on the diseased part. In the first case it is through the law of the contraries, and in the second through that of the similars. Notwithstanding, therapeutically the similars do better than the contraries, and dietetically these latter do better than the former.

The natural agents—cold, hot, moist, and dry—act on our organs and tissues as follows: the cold by contracting; the hot by dilating; the moist by relaxing; and the dry by straightening.

It is especially in hot countries that acute and hepatic (liver) disease develop easily. The hot air of these countries dilating the vessels causes in them an increase of blood, and consequently the liver is congested. Hence the frequency of these diseases in those countries. The same cause produces the acute diseases. And while hot countries give way to the acute and hepatic diseases, cold climates give way to the tedious and chronic diseases.

The same order of things occurs equally in temperate climates where the seasons are divided in two curves: first, the hot curve from March 21 to September 23; second, the cold curve from September 23 to March 21.

Yet, whether the winter instead of being cold, has been hot or tempered, the spring assumes this winter's abnormal hot or tempered influence on the humours, and gives way to the leucophlegmatic diseases coming out of a decrease of red globules in the blood. On the contrary, whether the winter was cold and normal, the spring's diseases are then freely inflammatory as the red blood was increased during winter's cold.

It is to be noted that spring's complaints are more acute and lethal than autumn's which are more tedious, longer, and leave some grievous *sequelae* withstanding the therapeutical measures.

Chapter II

The Heavenly Bodies and Their Influence

In the hands of Providence, man and things, willingly or not, are wonderful instruments which she contrives to use to her worthy ends.—Silvio Pellico

The law of universal gravitation which draws the bodies toward the center of the earth is also the law which governs the celestial bodies, maintaining them in equilibrium and giving them the impulse of the motion, of which they are animated. Hence their influence upon each other, the zodiacal belt, the earth and earthly matters.

On the other hand, the Moon, who is our nearest neighbour, and gravitates around us, assumes through the Sun and the planets a potentiality which she transmits to our planet conjointly with her own.

What is curious is the whimsicality of the phenomena produced by the Moon, i.e., the vigour and exuberance acquired by the trees, the capillary bulbus, the plants when the trees and the hair are cut, and the seeds are sowed two or three days before the

Full Moon; the turf which is destroyed by the chemical rays of the Moon; the crustacea gaining flesh with the Moon's increase, and losing it with her decrease; the human body augmenting in weight of one or two pounds during the Moon's growth, and losing them in proportion as she approaches of the last quarter, *(Sanctorius)*; the entozoons, the scabs becoming more burstling at the Full Moon; the skin diseases relapsing according to the lunar phases, and the itching becoming worst at the Full Moon; the fits of the nervous affections are more frequent toward the New and Full Moons (Dr. Lombroso); dreams and nightmares occur rather forty-eight hours before the Moon's perigee, when the Moon is about an hour high; pains occur in various parts of the body at the Moon's perigee. Besides, the goitre diminishes more or less during the lunar decrease, and the following treatment of this ailment is based upon this fact: "Cut a sponge in slices as large as a finger, broil them at the name of a waxlight, so as their middle becomes brittle; reduce the whole to powder, and three days before the New Moon, put two drachma of this powder in a bottle with a pint of rain or river water; cork well and keep the bottle in a cellar, taking care to agitate it once a day.

"Three days before the Full Moon, begin the cure, which consists of a spoonful of the remedy, to be taken morning and evening. So the most part of the bottle is used during the lunar decrease. The action of this medication is certain, and may easily be proved." (Dr. Goullon)

And the flow and ebb follow everywhere the Moon's motions. The great tides take place one day and a half after the New and Full Moons. When the Moon is New or Full, there is high water morning and evening, and when she is at her first and last quarters, there is low water.

As to the weather, it varies at the quarters of the Moon. So it rains mostly toward the second and third day of the first quarter, and the second or third day of the Full Moon than at any other epoch of the Moon's month.

The wind almost always changes at a New Moon.

The Athenians always married at the time of the New Moon; astrologically, this is the very best time to marry.

The Moon forms a conjunction with each planet once a month.

The cosmic, telluric, and meteorological perturbations, which are produced when the magnetic currents crossing the Earth in form of S from one pole to the other are actioned through the stellar influences, cannot fail to cause intransical modifications in the elementary qualities of the beings and things, and hence the genesis of multiple but periodic phenomena, because these influences are called for to be renewed at fixed epochs. So the twelve months of the year are not only unlike between them, yet differ of each other by a peculiarity owing to each one. Beside the fact that the seasons are antagonistic between them, the Sun in its apparent annual course abiding during a month in each zodiacal sign, influences this latter at times in one manner, and at times in another, but never in the same manner; hence, the differences of the months. So March of one year will have more similarities with March of the following year, yet still be distinct from one another. That is because the Sun entering Aries again marks the spring (March 21) and carries with itself not only the most part of the effluxions fixedly characterising the seasons, but yet those of the astral configurations varying each year.

The Sun does not occupy nearly the same point in the heavens, but at the end of a period of eighteen years *(Lalande)*, or more accurately at the end of thirty-six years.

This period of thirty-six years responds to the ancient's planetary cycle where the Sun and the Moon are considered as planets for the sake of calculations. This cycle is divided in seven circles, each one being ruled by a heavenly body which gives to the year of which it is the ruler its type and characteristics, especially at the point of view of the seasons and the earthly matters and environment.

Here is the cycle of Mars, beginning with 1909 and extending to 1944, inclusive:

Cycle of Mars 1909-1944

Circle of:

Mars	1909	1916	1923	1930	1937	1944
Sun	1910	1917	1924	1931	1938	1945
Venus	1911	1918	1925	1932	1939	1946
Mercury	1912	1919	1926	1933	1940	1947
Moon	1913	1920	1927	1934	1941	1948
Saturn	1914	1921	1928	1935	1942	1949
Jupiter	1915	1922	1929	1936	1943	1950

So, in a general way:

Mars: Characterizes a year with paroxysmic harshness of seasons (action and reaction), sudden and violent storms.

Sun: Tempered, rather warm year.

Venus: Tempered, agreeable, with warm showers.

Mercury: Windy, moist, variable.

Moon: Cold, moist, cloudy, transient.

Saturn: Cold, gloomy.

Jupiter: Cloudy with clear spots, transient showery, windy.

It is, however, not to say that the year ruled by such or such one of the heavenly bodies will necessarily show its type. The planet ruling the year only marks its possible constitution and character, which vary according to astral configurations presiding to the year's course. These latter alter the sunspots and so produce the terrestrial phenomena.

Here is a scheme of the solar latitudes as they are established by Professor Corrigan, an authority in the matter.

Thus, he proves that at the latitude of 5° north and south, the sunspots are engendered through Mercury's action on the Sun; at the latitude of 6° through that of Venus; at the latitude of 7° through our double planet, the Earth and Moon's action; at the latitude of 13° through Mars; at that of 48° through Jupiter, etc., and these spots have a more or less intensity and extension, according to the plants. So Mars causes a heavy band, Jupiter an immense band of monster spots, and Saturn makes large spots.

The sunspots have a periodicity of eleven years and forty days in average, but they are not less suddenly produced between the periodical intervals. This phenomenon is attended by a considerable atmospheric pressure, which at times raises the barometer up to thirty inches, and occasions frequent and sudden variations in the temperature of the upper atmosphere, which, entering in conflagration with the warmer atmospheric stratus of Earth's surface, give way to an abnormal production of static electricity (fiictional). Hence, perturbations in the telegraph transmissions, spontaneous explosions, earthquakes, etc.

It is observed that the great Jupiterian period of sunspots is of 27.36 days, corresponding to the lunar sidereal revolution of 27.32 days Further, it happens that on these Jupiterian periods the Sun, Jupiter, and the Moon are in conjunction.

And the Rev. R. Hicks says: "All our forecasts are based upon astronomic changes and conditions. There could be absolutely no such thing as weather and changing seasons if astronomic causes did not lie behind them, and weather and seasons would always be the same if there were no changes in the astronomic conditions out of which they sprang; and if the Earth and Sun were the only astronomic causes behind the storm and weather problem, it is clear that the same kind of storm and weather would prevail at the same time every year, as the physical relations of the Earth and Sun do not vary a hair's breadth of the same days for generations. And why all this perpetual change and variety? Is it all mere matter of accident or chance? For nearly half a century we have contended that every member of the solar system not only performs its functional part in the astronomic and physical equilibrium of the whole, but in the nature of the case must be also a factor in the meteorological conditions and results on our own and every other planet in the system. Heat, magnetism, and electricity inevitably result from the sudden stoppage or restraint of great force, while these forms of force disappear in proportion as they are converted into the form of motion. Hence we find our Moon contributing its part to the changes of temperature, the rise and fall of barometric pressure, the drift and changes of wind currents, and the minimum and maximum of magnetic and electrical potentialities, all these being the elements out of which arise storms, weather and earthquakes."

And as *mens sana*, healthy spirit, compels *corpore sana*, healthy body, so the astral configurations altering the terrestrial, electric, and magnetic currents, the temperature, the weather, briefly the earth's intrinsical constitution, affect the environment, and consequently the physical state of the newborn, principally at its conception, and subsequently at its birth, imprinting to it the mark or tone of its gamut of life.

Still, some twins differ physically and psychically, one from another. In such case it is sure that one of them was conceived prior to the other, and the proof of this is found in their (six pounds at term, and four pounds at eight months), which sensibly vary when the conceptions are not simultaneous, and whether the confinement takes place almost at the same time, it is because one of the foetuses being at term forces away the other one, which is not at term, but at eight months. The anticipation between the two conceptions is not less from a few days to one month. On the other hand, the conception point's stigmata or influences often prevail upon birth. I can cite twins born of a creole family. One of them was thoroughly of the complexion of its parents, but the other differed. It was obvious there were two conceptions, one before and the other just after the catamenia.

Chapter III

The Zodiac

*Sun Aries, Taurus, Gemini, Cancer, Leo, Virgo; Libraque,
Scorpius, Arcitemens, Caper, Amphora, Piisces.—Ausune*

The twelve constellations which are in the neighbourhood
of the Equator, and each of which comes to the meridian two
hours apart, have been called zodiacal, because they form around
the Sun a belt, 17° in width, which was called the zodiac, and
through which the planets revolve in a time and movement appropriate to each one.

The Earth equally runs over this zodiacal belt, which it di-
vides into two equal parts, through the orbit it describes around
the Sun. This orbit constitutes the ecliptic. As to our satellite,
the Moon, it evolves a fast movement around our planet, the
Earth, passing through all celestial longitudes in nearly twenty-
seven and a half days (sidereal revolution), and the Earth in its
movement of translation around the Sun carries with itself the
Moon. So this latter follows the ecliptic described by the Earth
around the Sun.

Still, the Moon through the movement around the Earth,
stands at times below and at times above the ecliptic in two
points, which are called Nodes. The North Node forms the

Dragon's Head, and the South Node the Dragon's Tail.

The Moon has also a rotatory movement upon her axis, offering the peculiarity of being of the same duration as her movement of rotation around the Earth.

The twelve constellations have not the same extension between them. On the contrary the twelve signs forming the zodiac are divided into equal parts of 30° each. The signs and constellations bring the same appellations.

The signs of the Boreal Hemisphere are: Aries, Taurus, Gemini, Cancer, Leo, and Virgo. The signs of the Austral Hemisphere are: Libra, Scorpio, Sagittarius, Capricorn, Aquarius, and Pisces.

These signs progress from the left to the right, i.e., the Sun through its apparent motion runs over them from Aries to Taurus, from Taurus to Gemini, etc., while in sequence of the precession of the equinoxes, the equinoctial point (March 21) goes backward in the zodiac of one sign every 2,160 years.

This point was formerly in the sign of Aries, i.e., in the constellation bearing the same name; but through the precession of the equinoxes it now responds to the stellar group Pisces. Nevertheless, it is quite correct to say that the Vernal Equinox takes place at the sign of Aries.

And in fact it must be so because whether the constellation Aries changed, the sign Aries did not, and the Vernal Equinox has always its ingress in the zone of influence betrayed by the node Aries occupying the 0° of the celestial longitudes.

So the constellations are not to be confounded with the signs, as neither the former nor the latter are to be confounded with the houses constituting another heavenly division which is wholly astrological.

Thus, the twelve signs of the zodiac form the zodiacal zones of influence and occupy fixed places on the zodiac, as is shown

The Zodiac

on the following figure.

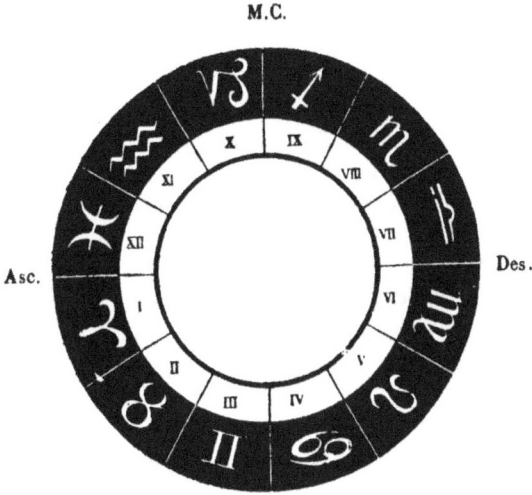

M.C.

Asc.   Des.

Each one of these zones operates on a part or organic system of the body with which it will be dealt further.

I maintain the fixed disposition of the zodiac as it perfectly adapts to the purpose of the heliocentric standpoint of astral science, as well as that of the solar-lunar's.

It may be noted that the node Aries of the zodiac constitutes the vital point of the economy on which depends nature's rhythmical operations. It is the east, it is the spring, it is the beginning of life and things, and in the animal economy it equals the Great Sympathetic.

Yet the true rulership of the general astral influences as to our planet, the Earth, pertains to the planetary system. The signs by themselves do not interfere directly with this action as they constitute but the notes of the Universe's harmony, entering in vibration through the planetary influx which action them, and consequently the Earth, its beings, and things. In fact, the Sun occupies the center of the planetary system, as it does the nucleus in the cellular system of beings, where it occupies the center of the cell, and both constitute the members of some algebraic equation, where the X gives way to the same positive quantity, *the life*.

On the other hand, it is obvious that the Moon, by her neighborhood to the Earth and her fast motions and variable potentialities, constitutes the "*Malaxator*" of the solar and planetary actions on the terrestrial matters, as Mercury does in regard to the Sun.

In further applications to medicine of the astral data. I will treat of heliocentric and solar-lunar systems, as according better with physiological and pathological purposes.

The zodiacal year begins March 21, under the node Aries, and finishes at the following March 21, under the sign Pisces. The civil day commences and finishes at midnight. The astronomical day begins and finishes at noon. It is counted from the first to the twenty-fourth hour.

In order to reduce the civil hours to the astronomical time, we must proceed as follows:

What is the astronomical time corresponding to a birth on January 25 at 10:00 pm? The civil day, having begun at midnight, the civil day of January 25 began at midnight. So 10:00 pm is equivalent to twenty-two hours after midnight. Now the astronomical day for the civil January 25, midnight, is January 24, plus twelve hours. So civil January 25, 10:00 pm, is equivalent to astronomical January 24 plus thirty-four hours, viz., astronomical January 25 at 10:00 pm (34 hours - 24 hours = 1 day + 10 hours), and civil January 25 at 10:00 am is equivalent to astronomical January 24 plus twelve hours plus ten hours equals twenty-two hours.

It must be noted that the Sun's daily motion is about one degree, and that of the Moon averages 13°19'.

Further, the zodiacal signs are subdivided into decanates, as shown below:

Sign	1st Decanate	2nd Decanate	3rd Decanate
Aries	Aries	Leo	Sagittarius
Taurus	Taurus	Virgo	Capricorn
Gemini	Gemini	Libra	Aquarius
Cancer	Cancer	Scorpio	Pisces
Leo	Leo	Sagittarius	Aries
Virgo	Virgo	Capricorn	Taurus
Libra	Libra	Aquarius	Gemini
Scorpio	Scorpio	Pisces	Cancer
Sagittarius	Sagittarius	Aries	Leo
Capricorn	Capricorn	Taurus	Virgo
Aquarius	Aquarius	Gemini	Libra
Pisces	Pisces	Cancer	Scorpio

Where each sign rules a zone of $30°$, these degrees proceed from March 22 to April 19 for Aries, from April 20 to May 20 for Taurus, and so on.

Each sign is positive and negative in rotation, beginning with Aries as a positive sign, Taurus as a negative sign, and so on.

Each zone of $30°$ is subdivided into three decanates. Each decanate is ruled by one of the three members of a ternary of the nature of the sign ruling the whole zone, viz., zone Aries equals ternary Aries, Leo, and Sagittarius (Hindu division of decanates).

The quadrant of Aries, Taurus, and Gemini of the circle rules the spring season and is positive. Cancer, Leo, and Virgo rule the summer season and are positive. Libra, Scorpio, and Sagittarius rule the autumn season and are negative. Capricorn, Aquarius, and Pisces rule the winter season and are negative.

The cell or ovum is the primarily departure of all beings in nature. The influence of two elements, the positive and the negative, is needed in order that the ovum may constitute a new being. These elements are ruled by the signs occupied by the Sun and the Moon at the impregnation moment of the ovum, but it is obvious that the principal part of the fecundation is incumbent to the Moon because the uterine gestation period is of ten lunar months (nine calendar months). The Moon each month accomplishes around the earth a whole revolution, so in ten months she evolves in the heavens 3,600°, i.e., 10 X 360° = 3,600°.

These later equal 273 days, resulting from the relative diurnal motion of the Moon, which is 13°10'35". Divided into 3,600, it equals 273 days[1].

The reduction of these days in zodiacal degrees results from the following rule of three. 365 days: 360° = 273 days: X. X. = 270°.

These 270° mark the zodiacal conception point, viz., the zodiacal point at which took place the impregnation of the ovum in the Uterus. So, to discover the solar sign and degree of the conception point, it is necessary to count back on the zodiac 270o, beginning with the birth's solar sign and degree.

As to the Moon's conception point, it results from that of the Sun's. In fact, the ephemeris indicates the lunar sign and degree corresponding to this solar point.

An example: Mr. X. is born September 16, 1870, at 4:00 am. The astronomical time equivalent to this dale is September 15 plus 16 hours. The Sun's 16 hours approximately respond to 0.66/100 of a degree, which are to be added to the solar longitude of September 15. Thus, solar longitude of Septembert 15,

---

[1]These 173 days are considered as the *average* time of pregnancy. I am rather inclined to anticipate that, deriving of lunar-solar combinations, they may be, in a normal and healthy confinement, regarded as the standard time of intra-uterine life of a child weighing six pounds at its birth, and as so relied upon for the calculation of the conception point.

1870 = 22°16' Virgo plus 0.66/100 of a degree for 16 hours = 0°40'. Total is 22°56' Virgo or 25° Virgo in round figures.

Now figuring back 270 from this sign and degree on the zodiac, we obtain for the solar conception point 23° Sagittarius, corresponding to December 15, 1869, *vide* ephemeris[1].

At this date the Moon was in 13° Taurus, and thus:
Sun's conception point 23° Sagittarius
Moon's conception point 13° Taurus

Referring to the Manilius secondary division, we have the secondary point Sagittarius for the Sun, and consulting the zodiacal scheme, we obtain for the 23° Sagittarius the decanate Leo. Summing up:

Secondary Points (Manilius)

Degrees	-	28	-	23	-	18	-	13	-	8	-	3
Degrees	30	27	25	22	20	17	15	12	10	7	5	2
Degrees	29	26	24	21	19	16	14	11	9	6	4	1
Signs	♓	♒	♑	♐	♏	♎	♍	♌	♋	♊	♉	♈

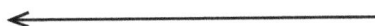

←

Sun's conception point 23° Sagittarius = Sagittarius
Conception secondary point 23° (Sagittarius) = Sagittarius
Decanate = Leo

and

Moon's conception point 13° Taurus = Taurus
Conception secondary point 13° (Taurus) = Leo

Hence, the following formula[2]:
Sun = Sagittarius + Leo
Moon = Taurus + Leo

---

[1]If the Moon is transiting, then it would be requisite to take account of the hour of birth.
[2]So difficult labour, necessity to recourse to forceps, etc., are but a sequel of Nature's working forces.

So it is not the newborn but the embryo that directly inherits the ancestral qualities which presided its conception time, and the newborn which at its birth's instant forms a quite new *unity* in the ranks of humanity, partakes of this very moment's environment, which endows it with its entity.

Still, at the medical standpoint the conception point must prevail upon the birth time, although this latter may often be subservient to the former, as "Nature makes all it needs in order that the native be born under celestial analogies in accordance with those of his breeds. (*Flambart*) Thus the arduous problem of the necessity to discover the conception point may be supplied if not entirely eliminated.

As to the infinite variety of beings, essentially differing between them, it necessarily results from the ancestral qualities not evenly distributed amongst the sperms and the ova. (Weismann)

Chapter IV

Airs, Waters and Lieus

Oh happy he that can the knowledge gain.
To know th' eternal God made nought in vain.—Culpeper

We owe to the genius of Hippocrates for having authoritatively dealt with this subject, which constitutes the stepping stone of the biological science. In fact, without airs, no organic exchanges; without waters, no new cells; and without lieus, no life.

It is through the action of cosmic influences on the airs, waters, and lieus that these latter operate upon beings and things so that it would be easy to judge of them according to their astral signatures.

Indeed, each town, each country, and each being and thing are ruled by the radical influence of a zodiacal sign characterizing them.

Are not the vegetables of a region or zone different from those of another region or zone? Do they not acquire more or less virtues, according to their habitat?

The climate, the exposition, the winds, and the soil on which they depend are liable to the medium which is modeled by the ruling zodiacal sign. Again, says Culpeper:

"Near the sea many people live, and Seraphion *(Artemisia maritima)* grows near them, and therefore is more fitting for their bodies because nourished by the same air; and this I had from Doctor Reason. . . .

"Lastly, it is known to all that know anything in the course of nature that the liver delights in sweet things, if so, it abhors bitter; then if your liver be weak it is none of the wisest things to plague it with an enemy."

Night air and moonlight are noxious, and they are especially so for producing malaria and miasmatic ailments. That is because through night's vegetal exhalations and diverse emanations the day's heat has not absorbed, and the air, by the prevalence of carbonic acid and the chemical action of the Moon's rays, becomes deleterious.

On the other hand, all in creation, from the smallest sand of the ocean to the tree of our forests, is endowed of caloric, electricity, radioactivity, etc. Yet, these forces are hidden. Nevertheless, as soon as on the Earth's surface or in its complexion there takes place a *friction*: winds, tempests, etc., are the result; a *decomposition*: moisture and fermentation are produced; a *trituration*: atomical and molecular separation or crushing is the result; a *kalalysis*: the osmosis is produced from, for giving way to a *chemical dynamism*.

And it is through these phenomena that the stars bring their contingency of action upon the airs, waters, and lieus; consequently upon man coming out of the Earth: *Pulvis es et in pulverem reverteris.*

Besides, the world has issued from the chaos through the condensation of waters, and from the waters the new cell borrows its constitutive elements.

In April and November where Sun's action upon our planet is weaker, the death rates augment and between intervals of these months they diminish.

The continuous and catarrhal fevers grow worst toward sunset, and the inflammatory and bilious fevers toward the sunrise.

Fluxions, pains, and tumours follow also a solar periodicity. They increase in proportion to the Sun's declination toward the west.

In a normal year the acute diseases more often show themselves or become more severe at the vernal and autumnal equinoxes (March 21, and September 23) and they diminish in intensity or are going away at the solstices (June 22, and December 22).

Moreover, the Sun is the sole vital agent of the Earth, and, therefore, of our organism. It destroys the morbid germs, hence the vitalizing action of the day (electric). The Moon, on the contrary, keeps them up and favors, hence the deleterious action of the night (magnetic).

Notwithstanding, these, as well as the astrometeorogical considerations, as to their relation from cause to effect, apply so far as man has not interfered with nature's works, such as clearing of woods, opening of an isthmus, etc.

Besides, the culture, especially the intensive one of the soil, modifies its qualities and properties, and a same plant differs in virtue according to its cultivated or wild state, as it differs also of virtues when it is transplanted in any other soil but its own. The same is as true for animals. The efforts made to acclimate at the Angora she-goat at the Cape of Good Hope produced almost negative results. The she-goat was pleased with the climate but its wool was modified.

This proves that we must be extremely cautious in uttering a final and absolute judgment because things good in certain conditions may be mischievous in some others.

Chapter V

The Synthesis of Constitutions and Temperaments

It is rare to encounter a person, who, in his early propensities, does not betray the point of his body and spirit, which would fail.—de la Rochefoucauld

As already stated, the constitution must not be confounded with the temperament.

The constitutive elements are those which preside to the formation of all beings and things, and are: oxygen, carbon, azote, and hydrogen. As we have seen, they respond to the ancient's elements: fire, earth, air, and water.

It is true that chemistry has not yet arrived to decompose the elementary bodies; that is not a sufficient reason for excluding the *Unity of the matter*. In fact, it would hardly be understood that Nature has some laws for certain bodies, and some others for certain other bodies, when the three kingdoms of Nature are indiscriminately subsidiary to the same forces: electricity, heat, light, magnetism, etc.

Still, new views in chemistry allow us to catch a glimpse of the *Unity of the matter.* So when some consider the colloidal state as marking the separation line between organic and inorganic bodies, some others such Ramsey and Berthelot, more and more restrict it through their experiences of transmutation.

The zodiacal signs, classified in their natural order in three sections of four signs each, present the following four *ternaries,* yielding each one to a dominant element:

First ternary: Aries, Leo, Sagittarius; fiery; equals oxygen

Second ternary: Taurus, Virgo, Capricorn; earthy; equals carbon

Third ternary: Gemini, Libra, Aquarius; airy; equals azote

Fourth ternary: Cancer, Scorpio, Pisces; watery; equals hydrogen

And the zodiacal circle containing the twelve signs is composed of the four quadrants:

First quadrant: Aries, Taurus, Gemini

Second quadrant: Cancer, Leo, Virgo

Third quadrant: Libra, Scorpio, Sagittarius

Fourth quadrant: Capricorn, Aquarius, Pisces

The first quadrant is formed of:

The fiery element; oxygen; Aries

The earthy element; carbon; Taurus

The airy element; azote; Gemini

The second quadrant is formed of:

The watery element; hydrogen; Cancer

The fiery element; oxygen; Leo

The earthy element; carbon; Virgo

The third quadrant is formed of:

The airy element; azote, Libra

The watery element; hydrogen; Scorpio

The fiery element; oxygen; Sagittarius

The fourth quadrant is formed of:
    The earthy element; carbon; Capricorn
    The airy element; azote; Aquarius
    The watery element; hydrogen; Pisces

So each one of these quadrants contains in itself three different elements, plus a fraction of the following quadrant's first element. These groupings give way to the cellular modifications responding to the following constitutions:

1. Bilious; oxygen; carbon, azote, plus a part of hydrogen. It is ruled by the Sun and Mars.

2. Lymphatic; hydrogen; oxygen, carbon, plus a part of azote. It is ruled by the Moon and Venus.

3. Sanguine; azote; hydrogen, oxygen, plus a part of carbon. It is ruled by Jupiter.

4. Nervous; carbon; azote, hydrogen, plus a part of oxygen. It is ruled by Mercury and Saturn.

In order to apply upon these data the individual constitution, let us proceed by an example. Mr. X's map where the Sun's sign of nativity (Capricorn) occupies the first zone or node of Aries, and the Moon in Taurus occupies the fifth zone of Leo.

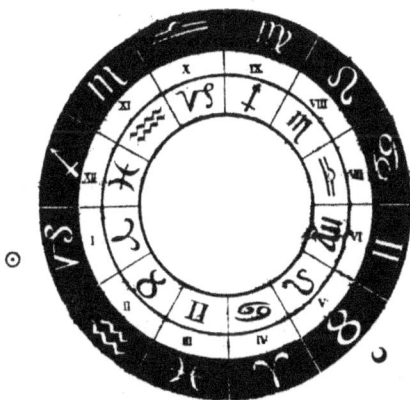

Thus:

Capricorn and Aries
Taurus and Leo
Gemini and Pisces

plus a fraction of Aries and Cancer from the first quadrant characterizing the individual constitution and where:

Capricorn equals carbon
Aries equals oxygen
Aquarius equals azote
Taurus equals carbon
Pisces equals hydrogen
Gemini equals azote

plus a fraction of Aries equaling oxygen, and a fraction of Cancer equaling hydrogen.

Summing up these elements, we obtain:

Oxygen: 1 and a fraction
Carbon: 2
Azote: 2
Hydrogen: 1 and a fraction

To which, adding the Moon's signs elements, i.e., Taurus equals carbon, and Leo equals oxygen, we have:

Oxygen: 2 and a fraction
Carbon: 3
Azote: 2
Hydrogen: 1 and a fraction

Hence:

Constitution = carbon, oxygen, azote, and hydrogen.

As there is no equality among these proportions, it needs to dissociate their principal constitutive elements as follows:

1. Carbon, which responds to the first constitutive element of the nervous constitution.

2. Oxygen, which responds to the first constitutive element of the bilious constitution.

So the individual constitutional synthesis presents as bilious-nervous and it partakes of Mercury, Saturn, Sun, and Mars, i.e., Mercury and Sun physiologically, and Saturn and Mars pathologically, as we will see further.

It must be noted that the liver is the "burner" of the economy, and the bile a combustion product.

On the other hand, the temperaments issuing of the constitution may be easily shown, although often they be mingled together. It may be said that they are the reflection of the constitution.

The typical temperaments are outlined below.

Lymphatic Temperament

The body is cold to the touch, and it is characterized as:
   Character: timid, distrustful, wavering, feeble, more stubborn than resolute, obliging by mania or self-esteem.
   Complexion: lax, fatty, and puffed.
   Eyes: grey or blue clear, little animated.
   Face: pallid or natural white.
   Forms: rounded.
   Gait: sluggish, listless.
   Hair: flaxen.
   Pulse: slow, soft, and flexible.
   Skin: smooth, white, veined of imperceptible thin, slowly growing downs.
   Stature: short and round.
   Teeth: large and coarse, broad rather than long; flat and badly shaped; regular in alignment; arch nearly semi-circular; opaque and muddy shade; they lack of character.
   Veins: narrow and profound.

It is among those of this temperament that one finds these honest clerks who wait for hours in an antichamber, or who work in an office during eight hours without moving. It is not because they are fond of working, but because they dislike any motion. They are sober (want of appetite) and chaste (want of sensual need), yet they do not despise altogether neither the table nor the pleasures. They are fond of all that does not necessitate the spending of a sum of energy.

> Diseases: These are, in a general way, chronic, affecting the glandular system: scrofula, scurvy, catarrhs, diarrhoea, ophthalmias, worms, cutaneous ailments (impetigo, eczema). They lack of reaction and present a low rate of fever so that they are difficult to come to resolution.
>
> Convalescence: Slow.
>
> Regimen: Substantial alimentation, dry, aromatic; fermented spirituous drinks, bitters; hard exercises, dry frictions of the body; abstention of prolonged baths.
>
> Climateric Conditions: Vivid air, hot countries and hot seasons.
>
> Accessory Measures: Dry 1 pound sweet orange peels in a shady place or in a drying stove. Let them steep during three days exposed to the rays of the sun in summer, or upon the chimney in winter in 2 pints good red wine. Let them dry up shady and keep for use. Chew some on the morning fasting. Enema with bran-water and a little mercury weed honey, and if this latter not to hand, use instead of, an infusion of chervil with an amount equal in size to a nut of fresh butter.

Sanguine Temperament

The body is moist to the touch, and it is characterized as follows:

> Character: Vivid, prompt to be carried away but easily getting milder, cheerful, gay, merry, laughing briskly, affable, voluptuous, flighty and changeable, bold at need

and magnanimous.

Complexion: Neither lax nor firm.

Eyes: Blue.

Face: Pink with plump cheeks.

Forms: Supple.

Gait: Vivid agitated, graceful.

Hair: Nut-brown.

Pulse: Vivid, but uniform and full.

Skin: White with winding of long blue veins.

Stature: Well proportioned.

Teeth: Medium in size; well proportioned; most beautiful teeth of four classes; cream yellow color; close and regular, arch a rounded square.

Veins: Large, salient, blue.

Those possessing this temperament are fond of table, pleasures, joyfulness, flattering, gay songs, witticisms; unpretending to anything, they are fit for everything.

Diseases: Acute in general, deriving of plethora (repletion), as are congestions, haemorrhages, inflammation of lungs, headaches, quinsies, palpitations, insomnia. They may be severe, inflammatory, and affect the heart and the blood vessels.

Convalescence: Fast.

Regimen: Beef, mutton, veal, fowl, white fleshed game; refreshing vegetables of kitchen garden, little bread; drinks: old wine, with water; exercises: riding; not tiring works; intellectual labors; moderation in everything.

Climateric Conditions: Moist countries, not rich in light and electricity.

Accessory Measures: Drink but water and take an enema composed as follows:

A handful of *parietaria officinalis*, tops

A handful of *mercurialis annua*, the herb without the root

5 to 6 roots of *cichorium intibus*

30 flowers of *viola odorata*
Half an ounce of *senna officinalis*
Half an ounce of *polypodium vulgare*
6 pints of *aqua fontana*
4 ounces of *honey*

Drink after each evacuation a herb-tea appropriated to the temperament and two hours after, a meat broth. No restrictions as to breakfast or dinner.

This enema suits all temperaments and maladies except when there are exhaustion and denutrition. It may be used as preventive at each return of seasons, especially of spring.

Bilious Temperament

The body is hot to the touch, and it is characterized as follows:

Character: Energetic, generous, stubborn, choleric, agitated, disdainful of riches, indefatigable worker, fond or glory.

Complexion: Lean, yellow-brown, dead dusky; vigorous muscles.

Eyes: Bright, black, and salient.

Face: Olive colored, expressive, serene.

Forms: Lean, dryed, hard.

Gait: Brisk, anxious.

Hair: Black, plentiful.

Pulse: Quick, but a little weak.

Skin: Yellow-brown.

Stature: Middle.

Teeth: Angular, long rather than broad; color, a rich bronze yellow (dried corn); regular and close together; arch rather square due to prominence of canines; transverse ridges on labial surfaces.

Veins: Coarse.

Those of this temperament are engaging, gallant, amorous and frankly deceiving, jealous and changeable; hearty eaters by need; fond of society, of strong spirituous drinks, and are gifted of a great vitality.

Diseases: Acute and long, easily degenerating in chronic ailments, and are due to a functional trouble of the liver. They are easily prevented by a vegetable diet, a moderate use of acids (lemons), tepid baths, cold enemas, sleep, recreation, moderate pleasures. Toward fifty years, this temperament changes to nervous or melancholic.

Regimen: Mucilaginous and plain food, not heating: lean meat, rice, semolina, artichokes, cauliflowers, gumbo, ripe fruits; abstain from milk and eggs; drinks: old, good wine with water or only water; exercises: running, walking,continuous but not violent. Recreations.

Are contrary to this temperament: fasting and complete diet, hot air, night's work, strong wines, violent passions.

Climateric Conditions: Temperate countries approaching spring's and autumn's temperatures in summer and winter.

Accessory Measures: Take the zest of 2 lemons and put in 2 pints of fresh water. Let macerate 24 hours. To be used by sips, between meals, two pints a day.

Nervous Temperament

The body is dry to the touch, and it is characterized as follows:

Character: Piercing, thoughtful, liable to dread, sadness, anger, grudge, varying of will and desire, meditative.

Complexion: Smooth, furnished of very black downs.

Eyes: More or less brown.

Face: Pale, of leaden color, with hollow cheeks; sad, anxious countenance.

Forms: Thin members, fine lines, long and slender fingers,

Roman nose, straight chest.

Gait: Vivid.

Hair: Nut-brown or sometimes reddish, greasy and flat.

Pulse: Small, rare, hard.

Skin: Smooth and brown.

Stature: Tall, well set.

Teeth: Medium or small in size; long, conical and flat; very sharp cusps; thin cutting edges; pearl-gray or bluish (quite characteristic); irregular and disposed to lapping.

Veins: Coarse.

He who is of this temperament is a devoted friend and an implacable enemy. He brings to excess the contempt of all enjoyments not caring for life. Able to execute the greatest actions in good or in bad; desirous of all sorts of renown; enterprising and shy; irreligious and credulous; distrustful and silent; exacting and envious; greedy of power but disgusted when obtained, there are no sacrifices to lay on himself for attaining his aim. Occupied of the happiness of the human genus, unhappy himself, he renders unfortunate all those that surround him. Reduced to poverty and put to a stump bedstead, he dreams of capital, and waking up, he is more surprised than confused to be nought. His style is oriental (fastuous), his word figurative and metaphorical and his imagination always in search of an ideal world.

Diseases: The exhausted constitution of the blood due to the decrease of its red corpuscles and the increase of its serum, contributes to exagerate their character: insomnia, constipation, and diarrhoea, piles, neurosis (epilepsia, hysteria, etc.), irregular appetite, headache (clavus hystericus), tic douloureux, intermittent symptoms.

Regimen: Meat, fowl; refreshing vegetables of kitchen garden, spices, ripe fruits, honey and sugar, except in acidity of stomach; drinks: copiously, light white wine with water, cider with water, small beer, skim-milk, barley tea; moderate exercise: walking, riding, rowing, gardening; moderate intellectual labor. Tepid baths.

Climateric Conditions: Temperate countries. Too hot seasons are more harmful than too cold.

Accessory Measures: 2 ounces *polypodium sulgare* (radix) and 2 pints *aqua fontana*. Boil and add, enveloped in a small linen rag, 2 drachms *potassi carbonas*. To be drunk at will during 8 days.

It is a pity that the hygienic and dietetic rules set down nowadays are dictated, as Dr. Schofield says, for an impossible and non-existing being—the average man. These simply theoretical and abstruse—because the living being is not the dead matter—chemico-therapeutical roles and prescriptions did not serve but to give way to the faddist, this average being of the family and social life! Nature in its wisdom giving to each individual a special temperament showed that what may agree with one may not be so with another, and that each one ought to subdue himself to the exigencies of his temperament. Nevertheless, in diseases, the diet will be useful, but diet is neither fasting nor food fadding. The first is wholesome and consists in getting away all that is of difficult digestion, and in moderating the hunger, while the latter is harmful because it consists in abstaining from all food. The celebrated Dumoulin before dying gave his friends the following advice: "I leave after my death," said he, "two great physicians: they are water and diet." Indeed, water and diet may do wonders, the first dissolving the thickened humours, and the second forbidding the humours to be thickened. On the other hand, rest and sedentary life debilitate the digestive organs, while a regular exercise not pushed to excess, morning and evening, before meal times, stimulates them and eases the digestion. The sole valetudinarian will abstain of it. (Avicen)

In acute diseases, nature has traced the way to be followed by its suppressing the appetite, and exciting the thirst. Here, barley-tea; sugar and water; acidulated water with lemons or oranges or pineapples; couch-grass or yarrow herb-tea lightly edulcorated with liquorice or coffee at will is all that is necessary for bringing the pyrexia to its period of defervescency.

We must remember that man is omnivorous and that his cellular constitution necessitates and implies a mixed feeding. Besides, each people have their own cooking and hygiene suiting their national temperament. Thus, it would be unwise to establish universal hygienic and dietetic rules. Here also people ought to conform themselves to Nature's laws.

We must remember also that we are not called to live an ascetic life, as did our forefathers, and whether they thought of dying, we will, on the contrary, as Goethe advises, think of living: "The things man ignores the more are those which are the more obvious."

It must be noted that among our food and the therapeutical agents suiting the necessities of our organism, the most are hot and dry. Here is again a Nature's law proving that the stimulants, the tonics, etc., suit better the needs of the economy because life is but a continuous struggle against death, and death is the result of the prevalence of the cold element. Yet through the gradation of the temperaments we are anticipated on the means we will make use of, in raising or moderating the vital stimulus. Hence the need sometimes of stimulants and sometimes of counter-stimulants, the hot and moist substances being those suiting in every circumstance.

So a gravy soup, an excellent claret, and some fresh eggs are all that is necessary for putting up a debilitated body, and they are more useful and wholesome than the phosphated flours, lecithins, and the kindred products got out of the chemist's retort.

Chapter VI

Physiological Synthesis

Vita brevis. Ars longa. Occasio praeceps. Experientia fallax. Judicium difficile.—*Hippocrates*

The aphorism of Hermes—"What is below is like that which is above"—thoroughly shows the straight connection existing between the universe and man who constitutes the microcosm. That is to say, in Nature all links together, repeats itself, and recurs.

And as the Earth is formed by the condensed fluids, so the cell nucleus is formed by the protoplasma.

Thus, man may be considered as a mirror where focuses Nature's forces through his nervous frame, which by its vasomotor action on the vessels, has charge of the distribution and regulation of the organismic fluids, and acts on the cell of which he is constituted. Two nervous systems take care of the individual: they are the sympathetic and the central. The first is that which presides to the vegetative life, and the other to the life of relation.

Nevertheless, man is made up of the germ, i.e., ovum. The fecundation of this latter absolutely necessitates the cooperation of two elements, differing in their nature as it is with the positive and negative poles of a battery, similars repulsing and dissimilars attracting.

The ovum is at first but a unique cell, slicing afterwards in many others, making cellular colonies of diverse species, hence the epithelial cells, the embryonal cells, the sanguineous cells, the nervous cells, etc., each having to fulfill a special function in the economy.

But none of these cells may be constituted without the inorganic salts which are constitutive of the cells, and, says Dr. Molesehott: "Without a basis yielding gelatine there can be no true bone, nor true bone without bone-earth, nor cartilage without cartilage salts, blood without iron, nor saliva without potassium chloride." And the organism provides itself with the necessary elements needed in the earth and air. Nevertheless, it is to be understood that these materials are molecular and not ponderous.

As I have previously stated, to the sympathetic nervous system pertains the care of the individual preservation, and this system is under their solar action.

The Moon, on the contrary, rules over the intercellular fluids and the organic systems through which they circulate.

It is certain that the Sun and the Moon in their action on the Earth carry with themselves the cumulative action of the planets revolving in the ecliptic, and that, as guiding bodies of the Earthly matters, they largely suffice to explain all the physical and chemical operations threatening in the economy. The planets can possibly alter the potentiality of Earthly matters, but they do it through the Sun and the Moon, giving rise to the solar spots which play a prominent part in the production of electrical phenomena on the Earth, consequently on the human body, considered as a galvanic pile.

We are imbued with the idea that man makes Nature to obey to his purposes. It is true that she yields momentarily, but she is not long in resuming her rights. Like the branch of a tree, which bends to a strain, but recovers its upright position as the tension is released, and just as the strain is maintained, the tree becomes curved and it takes an abnormal direction so the patient treated in spite of Nature's way inherits a life of physiological wretchedness, because Nature will be helped but not coerced. And Nature does not proceed in her operations by bewildering: *Natura non facit saltus*.

So the Sun's and Moon's actions exercise on the human organism through the innervation of the ganglia and plexuses of the sympathetic nervous system, the Sun presiding over the vegetative life, and the Moon over the humoural changes interfering in the economy. Thus, in:

Aries: Through the ganglion of Ribes emerging at the basis of the cranium, and the carotid and cavernous plexuses, they affect the cerebro-spinal nervous system, the head and its dependencies, and give way to hepatic diathesis.

Taurus: Through the superior cervical ganglion and the pharyngeal plexus, they affect the Eustachian tube, the neck, the throat and their dependencies, and give way to renal diathesis.

Gemini: Through the middle cervical ganglion, the thoracic (spinal) ganglia, and the deep cardiac, post-pulmonary, and right coronary plexuses, they affect the respiratory system and the upper limbs, and give way to cranian diathesis.

Cancer: Through the fifth thoracic (spinal) ganglia and the left coronary, diaphragmatic, hepatic, splenic and gastric plexuses, they affect the digestive organs, the pleura, and their dependencies, and give way to cranio-abdominal diathesis.

Leo: Through the splanchnic ganglia, they affect the heart, the cardia, the upper part of the stomach, and the dorsal vertebrae five, six, seven, eight, and nine, and give way to cardiac diathesis.

Virgo: Through the splanchnic ganglia, the solar and mes-
enteric plexuses, they affect the lower part of the stomach, the
abdominal organs, and their dependencies, and give way to cranian diathesis.

Libra: Through the lumbar ganglia and the renal, aortic and
hypogastric plexuses, they affect the renal system, the hypogas-
trium, the small intestine, the bladder in infants, and the uterus
in pregnant women, and give way to renal diathesis.

Scorpio: Through the lumbar and the intestinal branches of
the solar plexuses, around the umbilicus, the hepatic, suprarenal, renal, haemorrhoidal and spermatic plexuses, they affect the
brain, the medulla, the genito-urinary system, the bladder, the
uterus, the large intestine, the rectum, the anus, and the ductless
glands, especially the pituitary gland and the basal ganglia, and
give way to hepatic diathesis.

Sagittarius: Through the ganglion impar and inferior hypogastric plexus, they affect the muscular system (and the heart,
the gastro-intestinal tunics, the bladder), the hips, and the
thighs, and give way to thoracic diathesis.

Capricorn: Through the peripheral nerves and the connective
tissue they affect the cutaneous, mucous, and osseous systems,
the knees, and the thighs, and give way to splenic diathesis.

Aquarius: Through the sanguineous system they affect the
nutrition of the tissues, the lymphatic system[1], the legs and the
ankles, and give way to splenic diathesis.

Pisces: Through the plantar nerves, they affect the fibro-ligamentous, synovial and respiratory systems, the feet, the os calcis
and the toes, and give way to thoracic diathesis.

As to the planets, their role consists in adding or subtracting

---

[1]The blood is composed: a. of red corpuscles (erythrocytes), b. white
corpuscles (leucocytes), and c. of a colorless flud that holds the corpuscles in suspension during life, or liquid sanguinis (serum).

from the Sun's and Moon's potentialities. Thus: Mercury adds or subtracts to the nervous influx; Venus adds or subtracts to the renal process; Mars adds or subtracts to the hepatic process; Jupiter adds or subtracts to the thoracic process; and Saturn adds or subtracts to the splenic process.

And these five processes constitute the basis of all organic and organismic changes and alterations undergone by the cell according to the zones these heavenly bodies occupy in the zodiac. In a particular way: Mercury presides to the cellular irritation and the periodicity; Venus presides to the cellular retrogressive metamorphosis; Mars presides to the sthenic process; Jupiter presides to the hypertrophic process; and Saturn presides to the asthenic process, and the stenosis.

As to the Sun and the Moon, they sum up these processes and manifest them: the first through cellular excitation and the second through cellular zymosis.

1. The left side of the body is ruled by the elementary quality: cold.

2. The right side is ruled by the elementary quality: hot.

3. The elementary qualities moist and dry alternate so that the twelve divisions of the body are once moist and once dry.

4. The head is hot and dry.

5. The feet are cold and moist.

6. The dry and moist of the left side of the body are more feeble (cold) than those of the right side (hot).

Indeed, the twelve zodiacal signs are positive and negative in rotation through one of their qualities, where the elementary qualities hot and dry and hot and moist are positive, and those cold and dry and cold and moist are negative. So the sympathetic nervous system commences with positive Aries (paracelsus cerebral pole) and finishes with negative Scorpio (paracelsus genital pole), both ruled by Mars. The peripheral sympathetic nerves and the blood (in its composition) are the first under negative Capricorn, and the second under positive Aquarius, both ruled by Saturn.

From which results:

1. Relationship between the head and the pelvic organs positive Aries and negative Scorpio.

2. Relationship between the head and the cutaneous system and nerves positive Aries and negative Capricorn, and negative Capricorn and positive Aries.

3. Relationship between the peripheral nerves and the blood negative Capricorn and positive Aquarius, and positive Aquarius and negative Capricorn.

4. Antagonistic action between cutaneous system and the pelvic organs negative Capricorn and negative Scorpio, and negative Scorpio and negative Capricorn. For instance, sweat increasing, the renal secretions decrease, and vice versa.

We observe further the connection of Pisces with Leo, i.e., of feet with heart (edema of feet in cardiac diseases); of Pisces with Aries, i.e., of feet with cerebellum (wakefulness by cold feet); of Capricorn with Libra, i.e., of connective tissue with kidneys (anasarca); of Scorpio with Aries, i.e., of supra-renal capsules and kidneys with cerebellum (disturbed sleep and uremic coma in kidney diseases).

Again, Scorpio and Libra are nervous signs having a special action on the cerebellum (vegetative life).

On the other hand, according to tile zodiacal dispositions, the intimate and peculiar connection between the diverse organic systems presents as follows; that is, it is to say that in a general way physiologically and pathologically:

The head Aries and its troubles depend on the plantar system

Pisces and the abdominal organs Virgo.

The throat Taurus and its troubles depend on the blood and lymph Aquarius and the abdominal organs Virgo.

The lungs Gemini and their troubles depend on the peripheral sympathetic nerves and circulation Capricorn and the abdominal organs.

The stomach Cancer and the heart Leo and their troubles depend on the muscular system Sagittarius and the abdominal organs Virgo.

The kidneys Libra and their troubles depend on the genital organs and the bladder Scorpio and the abdominal organs Virgo.

So the abdomen and the abdominal organs Virgo form, so to say, the algebraic common denominator of all our organic functions and diseases, and this physiological and pathological truth peremptorily results from the zodiacal inspection. So that purging and clystering in spite of Moliere's sarcasms, remain yet thorough curative agents in diseases, especially if the physician happens to appropriate the drugs called for through year's, season's, individual's, and moment's stellar data, and to combine them with a tonic diet. The discredit in which they fell is especially due to their indiscriminate use and abuse and the general tendency to confine the diseases to the diseased organs, rather than to consider the organic systems in affinity with them, at the exclusion of professional and traumatic diseases. In fact, any peculiar localized disease is but an effect of a remote cause. So *sublata causa tollitur effectus*. Hence the marvelous action of wet abdominal compresses in acute and chronic ailments, of onion cataplasms applied to the feet in the cerebral forms of fevers and ague, and the great usefulness, as preventive, of hot foot baths, simple or revulsive with mustard flour.

At a humoural point of view, the four seasons; the four lunar quarters, and the four divisions of the day are similar in character between them, and here as in the scheme of the human body, the cold rules the months, the lunar quarters, and the divisions of the day which are more feeble, and the hot rules those which are stronger. And here and there the dry and the most come in rotation.

It is during the hours of sleep that the second digestion takes place, the ileo-coecal digestion which is the most important: *Somnus labori visceribus*, and the sleep is more restoring from midnight to sunrise, and more quiet during the lunar last quarter. The digestion in general takes place in fifteen hours. That is the reason of the predominance of the lymph upon other organic humours.

In fact, strictly:
    9:00 pm to 3:00 am has dominion the lymph.
    3:00 am to 8:00 am has dominion the blood.
    9:00 am to 3:00 pm has dominion the bile.
    3:00 pm to 9:00 pm has dominion the splenic humour.

Yet the year, said a sage, is but a long day. In winter one may indulge to his appetite with confidence.

Nevertheless, the intensive living to which the struggle for life subdues man nowadays unfolds more and more the nervous bilious temperament, which is the attribute of the intellectuality.

I said elsewhere that the first zone or node of the fixed zodiac, ruled by Aries, was the chief point presiding over Nature's operations.

So it is because all the diathesic and morbid evolutions depend on the sympathetic nerves which emerge from the base of cranium and preside to the vegetative life constituting the sole vital operation of beings before and after birth. For Nature made, as justly says Dr. McIntyre[1], the very wise provision that

---
[1]*Homeopathic Recorder*, vol. XXIII, p. 310. Boericke and Tafel, Philadelphia.

man shall not be permitted to interfere with his own nutrition. So every function of nutrition--digestion, circulation of blood and lymph, secretion, absorption, assimilation, excretion--is directed and controlled by the sympathetic system ruling the rhythmical action in every organ of our body. And rhythm is the universal property of the living matter. Besides, this system is the balance wheel of the cerebrospinal nervous system, which presides to the life of relation, hence the action upon the organism of the psychical influences.

Thus some pathological states take place through the action of the cutaneous capillary vaso-constrictor nerves (nerve fibres): Saturn, ruler of Capricorn and Aquarius; Jupiter, ruler of Sagittarius and Pisces; and some others through the vaso-dilatator action of the central ganglia; Mars, ruler of Aries and Scorpio. So certain diseases go from outwards inwards, and certain others from inwards outwards. It is to be noted that the mucous frame is as well an outward surface, although it covers inward organs. This is the reason why of the production of fifty percent of our diseases by cold, and as says Dr. McIntyre: "All remedies indicated in purely acute diseases must begin their action at the peripheral nerves, and all remedies indicated in chronic diseases must begin their action in the ganglionic centres."

The psychical influences are either depressing or stimulating. The depressings, or negatives, are anger, anxiety, care, dispair, despise, fear or fright, grief, melancholy, sulkiness, suffering, tediousness.

And the stimulatings, or positives, are cheer, creed, desire, decision, energy, gaiety, faith, hope, joy, resolution.

The joy excepted, which sometimes may be harmful, the other psychical stimulating influences are wholesome and strengthening.

Again, the suppression of an organ and the resuming of its functions in spite of its suppression, proves the great solidarity existing between the different parts of the body.

Thus the peripheral nerves, which attain the cutis and the mucous membranes play a prominent part in the production of morbid manifestations. They are ruled by Capricorn dominant Saturn. So, red face, dilated pupils, dryness of the faucess, nausea, and vomiting resulting from irritation of the nervous terminations of the mucous membranes of the stomach, roseola, breaking up of an irritative profuse watery diarrhoea, etc., depend on, and although these symptoms rather pertain to acute diseases, the sub-acute and chronic ailments depend as well on them as on the central ganglia.

It is to be observed that a molecular trouble of inorganic salts that are constitutive ones of the organic cell may give way to a disturbance of the sympathetic rhythmical action and so interfere with the individual diathesic evolution or morbidity. Nevertheless, this disturbance does not take place but through the liver's functions, this latter being the combustion fireplace of the economy, and the innervation of the cell depends thereon, so that the chronic hepatitis is the lot of ninety percent of persons.

The altered sanguineous principles, whatsoever may be their origin—scrofulosis, tuberculosis, lues venerea, cancer, gout, rheumatism, etc.—trouble the liver and affect the great sympathetic. The same process occurs with the suppression of a natural or morbid flow or discharge, and many cardiac diseases, especially the stricture of cardiac orifices, are produced in consequence of the liver's troubles.

Thus, all the organic systems noticed by the signs perform the rhythmical action of the great sympathetic, and thereby establish the straight connection existing between the physical diseases and mind.

And this peremptorily results from the heavenly bodies ruling the signs as follows:

Saturn is ruler of Capricorn and Aquarius

Jupiter is ruler of Sagittarius and Pisces
Mars is ruler of Aries and Scorpio
Venus is ruler of Taurus and Libra
Mercury is ruler of Gemini and Virgo
The Sun is ruler of Leo
The Moon is ruler of Cancer

Aries, ruled by Mars, presides to the sympathetic nervous system, and Scorpio, ruled also by Mars, presides to the intestinal ganglia and plexuses ruling the internal and external humoural secretions. On the other hand, Capricorn, ruled by Saturn, presides to the peripheral nerves, and Aquarius, ruled again by Saturn, presides to the blood's distribution and circulation in tissues. So these four signs form a qualuor on which depend all pathological manifestations to which Mars and Saturn remedies oppose alone or in combination.

Besides, the organic orifices which have charge of the elimination of the physiological or pathological products of the economy—urethra, rectum, nose, mouth, ears and skin—are ruled by Scorpio, Taurus, and Capricorn. To the first belongs the principal excretory orifices and to the second the subsidiary ones. As to the third, it marks the preponderance for health of the cutaneous functions, as death ensues the suppression of the cutaneous breathing (cutaneous asphyxia).

Another point deserving our attention is the utmost importance of ductless glands in the production of physiological and pathological facts of the economy. These glands are under the dominion or Scorpio, ruled by Mars, which notices that they take place through the fluxion Mars of the organismic fluids into the cavities, the cellular texture, or the substance of parts.

The metastasis or shifting of a disease from one part of the body to another or to some internal organ is also an important pathological fact. The homology or the immediate relation existing between diverse organs, tissues, glands, etc. of the economy explains these hidden affections of which the origin is unsuspected but which surely depend on the suppression or ablation of a remote organ such as the tonsils, the ovaries, the mammoe, etc. And what is worthy to be observed is the straight relationship existing between the opposite signs of the zodiac, and the organic ailments affecting seemingly different systems.

These signs are:

Aries—Cerebro-spinal system opposed renal system—to Libra

Taurus—Cervical nerves, throat, neck, genito-urinary system—to Scorpio

Gemini—Respiratory system and arms, muscular system, etc.—to Sagittarius

Cancer—Digestive system, cutaneous system, etc.—to Capricorn

Leo—Circulatory system, sanguineous system, etc.—to Aquarius

Virgo—Gastro-abdominal system, fibro-ligamentous and respiratory systems, etc.—to Pisces

Hence:

1. Encephalic ailments, and renal ailments: Nephritis, diabetes, and insomnia. Uremia, and coma.

2. Throat affections, and genito-urinary affections: Lues venerea and ulceration of the throat.

3. Respiratory organs diseases, and muscular system diseases: Bronchitis, and rheumatism.

4. Gastric troubles, and cutaneous and mucous diseases: eczema, etc.

5. Cutaneous affections, and blood affections: Eruptive fevers, anemia, hydrohaemia.

6. Abdominal affections, and fibro-ligamentous affections:

Podagra, gout, etc.

Let us remember that in human and Nature's things, beside what we perceive, there is what we do not perceive, and that any phenomenon, any action, any law does not beget a sole effect, but many. Of these effects only the first is immediate, the others spread out in succession. They are not perceived. (Bastiat)

As to the medical practice which assimilates our body to a laboratory retort, it is obvious that, as says Strindberg, the organic chemistry is certainly not the chemistry of the living body, but that of the corpse after incineration. Indeed, may a palace be inventoried on account of the celebrated painters, pictures therein, but now reduced by the fire to ashes? Surely not. Then what about these fruitless and hypothetical physiological views against which rise even the innocent animals as man's physiology wholly differs from theirs? So a long experience and a diligent observation of Nature's facts can guide us across the maze of life which always will remain in its essence if not its manifestations, a closed letter for us.

Now let me expose some anatomo-homological points which will be of utmost utility in astral diagnosis. Here they are:

Bladder Scorpio—Trachea Taurus
Bronchi Gemini—Ureters Scorpio
Chin (beard) Taurus—Pubes (pili) Capricorn
Coecum Scorpio—Stomach Cancer
Ductless glands Scorpio—Ovaries Scorpio; Pituitary gland Scorpio; Spleen Scorpio; Supra-renal capsules Scorpio; Thymus Scorpio; Thyroid gland Scorpio
Glandular portion of the uterine cervix and of the prostates Scorpio—Tonsils Taurus
Heart Leo—Prostates Scorpio; Uterus Scorpio
Ileum Virgo—Jejunum Virgo
Jejunum Virgo—Ileum Virgo
Kidneys Libra—Lungs Gemini
Large intestine Scorpio—   Esophagus Taurus

Larynx Taurus—Prostates Scorpio; Testes Scorpio; Uterus
  Scorpio
Lip (upper) Gemini—Perinoeum Scorpio
Liver Scorpio—Pancreas Virgo; Spleen Virgo; Kidneys
  Libra
Mammary glands Cancer—Ovaries Scorpio
Mouth Libra—Uro-genital orifice Scorpio
Muciparous glands of the generative organs Scorpio—
  Salivary glands Taurus
Nasal orifice Scorpio—Rectum Scorpio
Esophagus Taurus—Large intestine Scorpio
Ovaries Scorpio— Mammary gland Cancer; Thyroid
  gland Scorpio
Pancreas Virgo—Liver Scorpio
Perionoeum Scorpio—Upper lip Gemini
Pituitary gland Scorpio—Ductless glands Scorpio
Prostates Scorpio—Larynx Taurus; Mammary glands
  Cancer; Thyroid gland Scorpio
Pubi (pili) Capricorn—Chin (beard) Taurus
Rectum Scorpio— Nasal orifice Scorpio
Salivary glands Taurus—Muciparous glands of the gen-
  erative organs Scorpio
Small intestine Virgo—Ileum Virgo; Jejunum Virgo
Spleen Scorpio—Ductless glands Scorpio
Stomach Cancer—Liver Scorpio; Coecum Scorpio
Supra-renal capsules Scorpio—Ductless glands Scorpio
Testes Scorpio—Thyroid gland Scorpio
Thymus Scorpio—Ductless glands Scorpio
Thyroid gland Scorpio—Ductless glands Scorpio
Tongue Libra—Glans clitoris Scorpio; Glans penis Scor-
  pio
Tonsils Taurus—Glandular portion of the uterine cervix
  and of the prostates Scorpio
Trachea Taurus—Bladder Scorpio; Urethra Scorpio
Ureters Scorpio——Bronchi Gemini

Urethra Scorpio—Trachea Taurus
Uro-genital orifice Scorpio—Mouth Libra
Uterus Scorpio—Heart Leo; Larynx Taurus

Physiological Synthesis

Chapter VII

The Theme

The stars do not compel, unless we are already inclined;
then they draw us to their nature; however, if we let
ourselves be guided by reason, they may do nothing; but
if we only follow our nature, they compel and do with us
what they are doing with the beasts.—Indagine

The theme is fundamental for the understanding of the astral science. Indeed, without a celestial map this latter would be a mere theoretical and fanciful science and would have no practical use.

Three systems serve to erect a map resuming the resultant of the astral influences on the Earth's things. They are the geocentric, the heliocentric and the solar-lunar.

The first, the geocentric, is based on the calculations of the planetary positions in the zodiac, according to the planets' longitudes as to the Earth considered central of the planetary system. It is the Ptolemaic system and in general use in every astronomical observatory in the world. The second, the heliocentric, is that which suits better to Nature's order of things, the Sun being central according to the Galilean planetary system. And the third, the solar-lunar, where the luminaries solely and geocentrically

are considered, and their action is corroborated through an esoteric planetary gamut, is the more liable to the medical matters.
I will deal with these two latter systems.

The heliocentric system, which is the natural system, may
be compared to the cellular system. In fact, in this system the
Sun is placed at the center of the planets as is the nucleus in regard to the cell. Both are animated with a vital stimulus, and the
one and the other behave by irritation, which the Sun partakes
of the straight neighborhood of Mercury gravitating around it
(geocentrically, not far from 16° to 29°, and the nucleus of the
protoplasma surrounding it. Hence:

Mercury
Sun = Irritation
Protoplasms
Nucleus = Irritation

In the heliocentric order of planetary succession, starting
from the Sun, Venus follows Mercury and she is the Earth's next
neighbor. To her pertains the fecundation, the reproduction of
species and last but not least the fermentation equaling nutrition
(Dr. Béchamp), which is at the bottom of Nature's operations,
and as Paracelsus says: "Nature pulls her processes by fermentation and this latter is produced by hot and moist."

Resuming this we obtain the formula:

Mercury
Sun = Venus Earth

i.e., irritation equals fecundation, otherwise fermentation (nutrition). It is evident that the ancients were thoroughly cogni-
zant of the relationship existing between the Earth and Venus,
i.e., the positive and the negative elements ruling Nature's laws
as it may be deduced by their symbolizing the Earth with the
inverted sign of Venus.

Another fundamental process of Nature is periodicity, i.e.,

the rhythmical action which is, as I already said, the universal property of living matter, and of which Mercury on one hand and our satellite, the Moon, on the other hand, have charge.

Hence, the ultimate formula:

$$\frac{\text{Mercury}}{\text{Sun}} = \frac{\text{Moon}}{\text{Venus Earth}}$$

which characterizes the physiological evolution of the cell ruled by the heavenly bodies going from the Sun to the Earth.

As to its pathological evolution, it is subdued to the planets starting from the Earth to Saturn, the only known to the ancients, and which are Mars, Jupiter, and Saturn, and from the conflagration of these with the physiological planets results the morbid state. So, Mars presides to the inflammatory process without alteration of tissues; Jupiter presides to the inflammatory process with alteration of tissues; and Saturn presides to the inflammatory process with degeneration of tissues.

That is to say our diseases are often of an irritative and congestive nature. They may frequently be inflammatory, but diseases with tissue alteration or degeneration would be more and more rare. So death should normally depend on the sequences of old age if we do not anticipate it by our violation of the natural hygienic rules.

And, in fact, these three processes cover all the forms of disease the cell is heir to.

We stated elsewhere that man from the moment of his conception is ruled by the great sympathetic which emerges from the basis of the skull, and presides to the vegetative life. So the first zone or node of Aries, which rules the cranium and the encephalon, constitutes the vital point of the economy on which depend Nature's rhythmical operations. The Sun intrinsically influenced by Mercury incites the organismic rhythm through the first zodiacal zone of Aries, and thus excites the nervous cell.

But as soon as its action is transmuted by Venus, a retrogressive metamorphosis of the cells takes place and gives way to the cellular congestion, and later on through the influence of Mars or Jupiter or Saturn together or separately takes place the cellular inflammation with or without alteration of tissues.

The Moon, as regard to the Earth, excites also, but differently, the organismic rhythm through the zodiacal zones she runs over, and gives way to the zymotic periodicity.

But all these phenomena are yet subdued to a molecular trouble intervening in the inorganic constitutive salts and intercellular fluids of the cell, and so affect the cellular innervation which depends on the direct relationship existing between the mind and body.

Now, is there a possible connection between hygienic matters depending rather on man and his habits and the astral data?

No, if there was an artificial hygiene; yes, if besides the artificial, there is a natural hygiene which results from the constitutional needs and as so, depends on the astral science.

In accordance with what was exposed above, the heliocentric system is peculiarly liable to the terrestrial matters, the Sun being central to the Earth's motion.

Thus, the erection of a heliocentric map is an easy matter. Let us trace a circle with twelve equal divisions figuring the signs, and suppose a nativity, viz., on November 14, 1883, at 3:00 pm. Referring to Yarma Vedra's or Fredrick White's heliocentric ephemeris, we set out for November 14, 1883, the following speculum coeli:

Mercury in Scorpio	Mars in Taurus
Venus in Sagittarius	Jupiter in Cancer
Earth in Taurus	Saturn in Gemini

As to the Sun, it is in the sign Scorpio.

Now referring to *Raphael's Ephemeris* for the Moon's longitude, we find for the above date at 3:00 pm: Moon 19° Taurus.

Physiological elements:
Sun = Scorpio
Mercury = Scorpio
Venus = Sagittarius
Earth = Taurus
Moon = Taurus

giving way to the physiological formula:
Mercury   Moon
Sun = Venus Earth

Pathological elements:
Mars = Taurus by birth
Jupiter = Cancer acquired
Saturn = Gemini acquired

i.c., of these pathologically threatened signs, only Taurus partakes of the physiological signs, so its maladies are by birth; the other two, viz., Cancer and Gemini's threatening diseases, are acquired.

Thus of this heliocentric chart resorts the following formula:

$$\text{♏}^{\text{♏}} = \text{♓} \; \text{♉}^{\text{♉}}$$

Substituting to the signs in exponent their planetary rulers, we get the formula:

$$\text{♏}^{\text{♂}} = \text{♓} \; \text{♉}^{\text{♀}}$$

But as Mars rules also Aries, and Venus rules also Libra, then:

$$\text{♏} \, \big|_{\text{♈}}^{\text{♂}} = \text{♓} \; \text{♉} \, \big|_{\text{♎}}^{\text{♀}}$$

This is the individual physiological standard formula.

As to the pathological standard, I observe that Taurus alone figures among the signs ruled in the map by the pathological planets and in the present case, it is done by Mars. Hence the formula[1]:

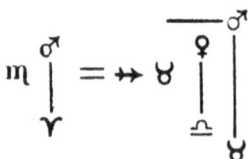

It forms the first step of diseases the subject is heir to, Mars.

Further, of the pathological planets, Jupiter rules Cancer, and Saturn rules Gemini. Hence, the following pathological formulae:

Second step:

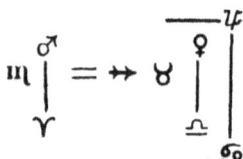

Third step:

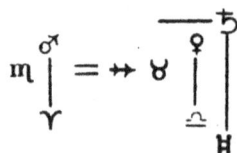

I will deal with the reading of this heliocentric chart in the chapter on the practice.

---

[1] The pathological planets in exponent mark the individual predisposition to some pathological evolution, and each individual manifests it according to his ancestral qualities.

As to the solar-lunar system[1], "it results from the mutual influences of the Sun and Moon in their relation with the zodiac because the Earth in its course into the zodiacal circle receives the solar rays transmuted through the planetary action on the Sun. This latter constitutes the seasons, the months, the days, etc., and its motion is steadfast although progressive in the course of the year. On the contrary, the Moon with her swift motions and her frequent relations with the zodiac, continually modifies and transmutes the solar influence, adding to it her own. Hence, two influxes, complementary between them, ruling Earth's things. The first slow, constant but progressive, monthly and daily duet of the Sun[1], and the other, rapid, transitory, variable, septenary, diurnal, and horary due to the Moon.

This solar-lunar system which synthesizes the astral influences through the luminaries is not only simple and more convenient, but yet more suitable to the medical matters. It has among many advantages that of eluding the need of considering the Sun and the Moon as planets for the sake of calculations. Still, for its being of a general application, as it is too restrained in its elements, this system needs to be completed. So we can practically take advantage of the peculiar esoteric properties ascribed by the Ancients to the planets.

Further, we notice that the signs of the zodiac can be considered as the ordinary notes of a keyboard, its first note being Aries and its last Pisces, and where the seven planets, in their esoteric order (Sun, Venus, Mercury, Moon, Saturn, Jupiter, Mars) constitute the diesis and flats: the Sun for Taurus, Venus for Gemini, Mercury for Cancer and so on. But in so doing, we consider the planets as exponents of the zodiacal signs, where they serve to

---

[1]Indagine, celebrated astrologer of 17th century, says: "I will seem audacious to undertake to do what was done by few before me (Eudoxus, Lyechtemberg, etc.) and deal with Natural Astrology. This latter was despised because it is simpler. Nevertheless, allow me, learned men, to ascertain that it is more faithful, and does not deceive us."

mark the physiological and pathological modalities subdued to each one, Aries excepted.

There is the zodiac in rest.

Should a nativity occur, then immediately it enters into activity vibrating at the diapason of the ruler of the solar sign (and of that of its decanate, if any) of the birth time, which gives the individual key or intonation to the sign Aries of the keyboard constituting the fixed zodiac.

Now, the Sun and the Moon come into play and occupy their respective astronomical places (as it results from the nativity). They give the measure and modulation to the individual melody which any one of us is called to play as soon as our births on this earthly planet take place. In fact, the Sun by its slow movement typifies the hour hand of the great clock of the Universe and marks the hours (measure), and the Moon by its fast movements presents the minute hand of this clock and marks the minutes and seconds (modulation). Elsewhere they cumulate and synthesize the conjoined planetary action.

So we have in our map an instrument which beats at the unison of that which constitutes the Universal harmony, and joins the macrocosm to the microcosm, i.e., the Man. And the Universal harmony results from the dynamics of the ondulation.

It is to be noted, as I already observed, that the spring's node Aries of the fixed zodiac constitutes for the animal economy the point of the great sympathetic whose ganglia and plexuses are distributed among the signs, Aries through Scorpio, the first eight of the twelve, the remaining four signs (Sagittarius, Capricorn, Aquarius, Pisces) denouncing the relation of some particular organismic regions with the sympathetic and cerebro-spinal nervous systems.

It is to be noted that the hour of nativity is necessary especially for the Moon's motions.

As to the individual vitality, it depends on nativity's celestial directions. So under the horizon (zones I to VI), it is feeble, and above, the horizon (zones VII to XII), it is strong.

The prognostication is resumed from the Sun and Moon's relative aspects. The principal aspects are the following and are either favorable or unfavorable:

0°	Conjunction	Favorable
60°	Sextile	Favorable
90°	Square	Unfavorable
120°	Trine	Favorable
150°	Quincunx	Unfavorable
180°	Opposition	Unfavorable

Among the zodiacal zones, seven have a physiological and pathological importance. These seven are:

1. Sun's zone, variable in its sign, but always occupying the fixed zone of Aries.
2. Moon's zone, variable.
3. Zone XII.
4. Zone XI.
5. Zone VI.
6. Zone VII.
7. Zone VIII.

Now for erecting a solar-lunar chart, let us consider the nativity which served us to illustrate the heliocentric system, with Mr. X, who was born November 14, 1883 at 3:00 pm.

According to the zodiacal scheme, the Sun occupies 21° Scorpio and Raphael's Ephemeris for the year 1883 at the above date and hour, gives 19° Taurus for the Moon.

Still, before going further with the reading of the map, I would like to point out that neither the Sun nor the Moon can be rulers of the birth's signs. In this case the ruler of the sign following the birth's sign becomes ruler of the birth's sign. So Sun

in Leo by birth will give way to Mercury ruler of Virgo following Leo, and the Moon in Virgo by birth will give way to Venus,
ruler of Libra, following Virgo. Again, the Moon or the Sun in
Cancer cannot give way to Sun ruler of Leo following Cancer,
but to Mercury ruler of Virgo. (Indagine)

On the other hand, the Sun staying thirty days in each sign
turns nearly one degree a day, and 360 degrees in a year. The
thirty degrees of each sign are divided in three equal parts of ten
degrees each, forming the decanates. The first decanate, one to
ten degrees, is ruled by the solar sign of the month; the second
decanate, from eleven to twenty degrees, is ruled by the second
sign of the ternary at which pertains this solar sign, and the third
decanate, from twenty-one to thirty degrees, by the third sign
of this ternary. Thus, Aries being, for instance, the first sign of
the decanate, Leo will be the sign of the second decanate, and
Sagittarius that of the third decanate. So, for the above nativity,
the significator of its chart will be Scorpio, where stays the Sun
from October 23 to November 22, plus Cancer, third decanate,
as from October 23 to November 14 inclusive, there are twenty-
one days or twenty-one degrees. This order of the decanates is
that of the Hindu method founded upon the triplicities. i.e.,
ternaries of the signs. Thus:

Sun in Scorpio decanate Cancer, viz:

    Mars, ruler of Scorpio   equal tonality or
    Mercury, ruler of Cancer   individual vitality

Moon in Taurus, viz:

    Mercury, ruler of Taurus   equal modalities subdued
                                  to the individual tonality
                                  or vitality

The Sun in 21° Scorpio, and the Moon in 19° Taurus are in
opposition between them, i.e., in adverse aspect, hence:

Prognostication: reserved.

On the other hand, in the above chart the esoteric planets: Sun, Venus, Mercury, and Moon occupy double zones, and Saturn, Jupiter, and Mars single zones. The first four are physiological and the three latter pathological. So the physiological state results from the organic systems ruled by Sun, Venus, Mercury, and Moon,which are represented by the following signs:

Taurus and Sagittarius for Sun
Gemini and Capricorn for Venus
Cancer and Aquarius for Mercury
Leo and Pisces for Moon

As in the above nativity the Sun occupies 21° Scorpio, i.e., the first zone; then, of the esoteric double planets those which are under the horizon will prevail. So the characteristic planets of this nativity will be:

Sun of second zone of Taurus
Moon of fifth zone of Leo
Mercury of fourth zone of Cancer

Further:

The twelfth zone of Pisces and Libra denotes the individual constitutional drawback.

The eleventh zone of Aquarius and Virgo marks the physiological changes or alterations undergone by the sanguineous system under the constitutional drawback of the zone twelve.

The sixth zone of Virgo and Aries indicates the pathological localizations resulting from zones twelve and eleven.

The seventh zone of Libra and Taurus denotes the changes or alterations undergone by the humoral, secretion of the economy.

The eighth zone of Scorpio and Gemini sums up the trouble or troubles supervening in the organism in consequence of the above stated conditions.

I anticipated that pathological planets were Mars, Jupiter, and

Saturn. Referring to the above chart, I notice that Saturn rules the sixth zone of Virgo, Jupiter the seventh zone of Libra, and Mars the eighth zone of Scorpio. Of these signs, the first. i.e., Virgo, presides over the abdominal organs, namely the liver, the vena portoe, the spleen, the small intestine, and the solar plexus. Thus our diseases always originate in the abdominal system, and hence the common and general use of beginning by deterging the *primae viae*, before instituting the treatment of any acute ailment. Besides Mercury, ruler of Virgo, betrays the action of the mind upon the body and vice versa, and the reflex nervous origin of the gastro-abdominal organs and troubles.

The second sign of Libra of the zone seven rules the renal system, i.e., the secretion of the waste liquid products of the economy, the kidneys constituting a filter through which pass these matters. Besides, its ruler Venus notices the fermentative (nutritive) and distillatory processes to which they are subdued in the economy.

Further, the third sign of Scorpio, ruling the genito-urinary system, the pituitary gland, and all the excretory processes of the economy, indicates Nature's way of getting rid of the organic waste matters (liquid and solid) whose elimination from the organism takes place:

1. Through the urines, of which the receptacle is the bladder.

2. Through the feces, of which the receptacle is the bowels. These latter are lubricated and aseptised by the bile, which thus regulates their daily physiological functions.

3. Through the nose.

Also, its ruler Mars notices the combustion or coction process to which these waste products are undergone in the economy. Hence the importance in diagnosis of the urine's and force's examination or analysis.

Thus these physiological and pathological facts and truths are exemplified in a wonderful manner by the astral chart and peremptorily prove the profoundness of the Hippocratic medicine.

Summing up:

Tonality	Mars in Scorpio and Aries
	Mercury in Cancer and Aries
Modalities	Mercury in Taurus and Libra
Prognostication	Sun opposition Moon in
	adverse aspect

Solar sign zones:
Libra and Pisces in twelve
Virgo and Aquarius in eleven
Leo and Capricorn in ten
Aries and Scorpio in six
Taurus and Libra in seven
Gemini and Scorpio in eight

Esoteric planet zones:
Sun in Taurus and Sagittarius in two
Moon in Leo and Pisces in five
Mercury in Cancer and Aquarius in four

Reading of the Chart

The Sun is in Scorpio and Cancer decanate, but it yields its potentialities to Mars and Mercury.

So the native's physiological and pathological standards proceed from Mars and Mercury. Thus his constitutional tonality will be hepatic Mars nervous Mercury, and manifests itself through the genito-urinary, hepatic, splenic systems, the large intestine, the coecum, rectum, anus, and pituitary gland Scorpio, which notice an insufficient elimination of the physiological excretory fluids and salts Scorpio in consequence of a defective innervation Mercury of the digestive organs Cancer. These troubles taking place in the first zone of Aries further confirm their nervous origin.

As to the constitutional modalities, they result from the Moon in Taurus and Libra, viz., Mercury in Taurus and Libra, the ailments the native is heir to, will involve the throat, the neck, the sub-maxillary glands, the pharynx, the mouth Taurus and affect the renal system (secretion) Libra. They may be irritative Mercury.

The prognostication (in chronic ailments) results from the aspect of the Sun and Moon. Here they are in opposition, i.e., in adverse aspect. So it will be reserved.

Thus the sole consideration of the Sun and Moon in a solar-lunar chart is mostly sufficient for judging a nativity at the standpoint of its physiological and pathological predispositions. Notwithstanding, a further accuracy may be obtained by viewing first the solar sign zones, and second the esoteric planet zones.

The zones twelve and eleven mark the humoural trouble's origin through the heredity Pisces and the blood's condition Aquarius. This trouble takes place through the renal system Libra and the gastro-abdominal organs, and the solar plexus Virgo.

The zones six and seven indicate the tendency of this trouble in localizing itself in the gastro-abdominal Virgo and renal systems producing, through the nervous sympathetic system's influx Aries, an affection of the throat, etc. Taurus.

And the zone eight betrays the ultimate phase of the constitutional taint which through the defective elimination of the excretory matters of the economy Scorpio may affect the pulmonary haematosis Gemini.

Further, the esoteric planets' zones, under the horizon, i.e., negative, show:

1. A lack of salivation (Taurus and Sagittarius Sun).

2. A lack of heat in lower extremities (Leo and Pisces Moon);

YEARS						ZODIACAL ZONES											
						I	II	III	IV	V	VI	VII	VIII	IX	X	XI	XII
61	49	37	25	13	1	♏	♐	♑	♒	♓	♈	♉	♊	♋	♌	♍	♎
62	50	38	26	14	2	♐	♑	♒	♓	♈	♉	♊	♋	♌	♍	♎	♏
63	51	39	27	15	3	♑	♒	♓	♈	♉	♊	♋	♌	♍	♎	♏	♐
	52	40	28	16	4	♒	♓	♈	♉	♊	♋	♌	♍	♎	♏	♐	♑
	53	41	29	17	5	♓	♈	♉	♊	♋	♌	♍	♎	♏	♐	♑	♒
	54	42	30	18	6	♈	♉	♊	♋	♌	♍	♎	♏	♐	♑	♒	♓
	55	43	31	19	7	♉	♊	♋	♌	♍	♎	♏	♐	♑	♒	♓	♈
	56	44	32	20	8	♊	♋	♌	♍	♎	♏	♐	♑	♒	♓	♈	♉
	57	45	33	21	9	♋	♌	♍	♎	♏	♐	♑	♒	♓	♈	♉	♊
	58	46	34	22	10	♌	♍	♎	♏	♐	♑	♒	♓	♈	♉	♊	♋
	59	47	35	23	11	♍	♎	♏	♐	♑	♒	♓	♈	♉	♊	♋	♌
	60	48	36	24	12	♎	♏	♐	♑	♒	♓	♈	♉	♊	♋	♌	♍

hence, nervous dyspepsia (Cancer and Aquarius Mercury).

Furthermore, man evolves upon his constitution so that in order to get the modifications undergone by this latter in life's course, it needs to revolve the zodiac, which goes back each year a sign, as can be seen in the preceding chart.

Thus, Scorpio occupying the first zone the first year, Sagittarius succeeding to Scorpio will occupy the same zone the year after, and so on. Nevertheless, the first sign of nativity, i.e., Scorpio in the present case will prevail in the zodiacal revolution, and so will do its decanate, if any[1].

It is to be observed that like the zodiacal zones, the heavenly bodies have also their fixed zones of influence which must not be confounded with their astronomical evolution. These planetary zones respond to the seven heavens of the ancients, of which each one corresponds to a planet, the seventh being that of Saturn, the sixth that of Jupiter, etc.

---

[1] The zodiacal revolution marks yearly the organs or orgasic systems which will in the course of life be hit by the individual diathesis, which does not vary. The critical year is the sixty-third for everyone. Critical years are equally every seven years after birth.

In fact, I remarked that a theme geocentrically erected does not, as the one I have just unfolded, answer to the study of the diathesis. In order to get the individual physiological or pathological cellular coefficient, the prognostication, etc., it deserves to be noted that the planets esoterically placed acquire a more peculiarly accurate meaning than those obtained astronomically.

Thus the signification of the zones six and eight remains unchanged in the esoteric map, when it varies in an ordinary one.

Besides, I remark that Mars geocentric often occupies zone eight when a lethality, precocious or not, threatens the subject, or it is in opposition to this zone. The same is observed with Saturn geocentric.

The synthesis of a theme is furnished by the sign occupying the diagonal of the zodiacal revolution. This sign constitutes the hypotenuse of a triangle, the sides of which are formed of the twelve zodiacal signs, beginning with the solar sign of nativity.

I will add that an astral chart, betraying the constitution or diathesis, the individual predispositions, etc., is not fit for adapting itself to the nosological entities but indirectly, as a morbid entity implicates a lesion, and this lesion did not take place but through a morbid evolution, and step by step, and as Paracelsus says:

> "It is absolutely true that stars and their influences inflict to men the most part of their diseases and make them enter into their body. However, they do not this either with violence nor ostensibly as it maybe perceived immediately. They do it slowly, insensibly, imperceptibly until the sickness results therefrom, such the oil distilled drop by drop which is only appreciable when there is a certain quantity heaped up in the vessel."

So it would be inopportune to depend on the astral influences for all that depends on man himself. In fact, he who eagerly eats is sure to catch an indigestion. Surely the stars are not interfering therein.

Reduced thus to its simplest expression the astral chart is in conformity with the antique traditions whose rules were established by the fathers of cosmogony. So it excludes the personal interpretation.

As to the physical, astro-meteorological, seismic or atavic and hereditary phenomena, they result from the astronomical facts and are founded on mere experience and observation.

Now a word on the determination of child's sex before the birth. It depends on the lunar influences. Indeed, it is observed that if the Moon was new among the nine days following the birth of a child, the next child which will be born will be of the same sex, and if the Moon was new after the elapsing of the nine days of birth of a child, the next child which will be born will be of a different sex.

The Theme

Chapter VIII

Pathological Synthesis

Physic without Astrology is like a lamp without oil.—
Culpeper

T wenty three centuries have elapsed since Hippocrates established the foundation of medicine, and his teaching is as true
nowadays as it was then. That is because Hippocrates based it
upon Nature's universal laws and observation. Indeed, in order
that a remedy may duly be applied, the physician, says he, must
have a knowledge of astrology. His therapeutics consisted in
Simples and Physical Agents.

Except for some notorious physicians who were illustrious in
antiquity, we must go back to the 15th century to encounter another genius deserving our admiration. This genius is Paracelsus.
Like Hippocrates and the Arabian physicians, he based his medical conceptions upon astrology, and made use of the chemical
preparations in therapeutics, and composed his *Arcana*.

Rademacher, in modern times (1772-1850), was his scientific follower and interpreter.

But to Hahnemann (1755-1843), modem medicine is indebted for the adaptation to medical practice of a natural law

permitting to attain the morbid causes through the effects. Indeed, his law of the similars is that of analogy and harmony, the therapeutical agent fit to produce analogous symptoms to a disease, necessarily yielding to the same morbid evolutionary course as the disease, to enable it to produce similar symptoms. Hahnemann thus confirmed the Hippocratic teaching and placed himself against the Nosological entities which are merely established on the effects rather than on the causes.

It is obvious that an organic lesion involves but an evolution of the constitution or diathesis. This diathesis we are heir to, from the moment of our conception, and is such, as sidereal, telluric, and cosmic conditions modeled it, at this very moment. It may be scrofulous, cancerous, tuberculous, etc.; yet we cannot recognize these diathesic drawbacks but through the individual theme and that of the parents.

The points to be considered in a solar-lunar theme, are the following:
1. The Sun's place marking the tonality of the vital force.
2. The Moon's place marking the modalities undergone by the same.
3. Zone XII characterizing the humoural alteration through fatality.
4. Zone XI betraying the blood's condition.
5. Zone VI betraying the morbidity.
6. Zone VII characterizing the secretory process through the kidneys.
7. Zone VIII betraying the prognostics.

And this gradation is that Nature follows in the evolution of her works, and responds to the diverse combination of the primordial elements. I already stated: *Natura non facit saltus.* Thus, health and morbidity result from the conditions of the abdominal organs through the fixedly dominated sixth zone of Virgo, ruler Mercury, consequently are under the dependency of the innervation betrayed by the solar plexus actioned in health through psychical stimulating causes, and in sickness through the psychical depressing causes. This sixth zone is, in the solar-lunar system, under the esoteric dominion of Saturn; hence, humoural secretions which whether physiological entertain the health, and whether pathological cause the morbidity. The humoural secretions are betrayed by the seventh zone of Libra, ruler Venus. This zone is under the esoteric dominion of Jupiter. The humours, not eliminated from the economy, repercuss on the organic system threatened by nativity (diathesis). They are noticed through zone eight of Scorpio, ruler Mars, and give way to the prognostics. This zone is also under the esoteric dominion of Mars. I will add that Scorpio presiding over the ductless glands of which partake the suprarenal capsules, the pituitary, the thyroid, the thymus glands, the genito-urinary, renal systems, the testes, the ovaries, etc., including the key of all physiological and pathological changes entertaining or threatening the life through the innervation of the sympathetic nervous system. That is the reason of the utmost importance of the organoleptic examination of the Urines which resume the morbid alterations betrayed by Scorpio and its ruler Mars.

The thymus gland disappears with the adult age. It must contribute to the growth of the body.

On the other hand, the nose plays a great role in many diseases: the fits of sneezing premonitory to asthma, the pituitary localizations of La Grippe, of hay fever; the epistaxis (bleeding of the nose) pathognomonic of enteric fever, etc., are under the dependency of the innervation of the pituitary gland and basal ganglia. Thus the great moral and physical depression, the troubles in diuresis and diaphoresis, the pyrexia, which are common to many ailments, unknown in their origin, often proceed from the pituitary gland's and basal ganglia's troubles. In fact, the pituitary gland's extract taken internally increases urination and augments the body's fat integuments, which are in accordance with the law of similarity. Further, the suprarenal capsule's extract is heroic in convalescence of diphtheria, scarlet fever, etc, as the suprarenal insufficiency is at the bottom of these complaints. Again, the urine sometimes reacts the albumen in spite of the healthiness of the kidneys. It is because the suprarenal fluid mingles in the urine.

I will incidentally say that Pisces' zone twelve of fatality indicates atavism and heredity. And curiously we observe that a sole humoural principle, proteiform in itself, is betrayed by Pisces ruling the fibro-ligamentous and synovial system and the feet (Podagra). That is arthritism which was called Psora by Hahnemann and which is peculiar to the omnivorus beings. So it depends on the individual disposition, and is not acquired through an outward cause like syphilis and sycosis. These latter may be grafted on the first and complicate it, but they do not result, as arthritism does from a natural law which is the organic need of beings for eating meat. "Man at his finest and most active period of life," says Dr. Forbes Ross, "was a hunter and hunters are essentially meat-eaters."[1]

The diverse signs which occupy zone twelve mark the form of arthritism according to the individual theme.

I willingly did not deal with death.

I will observe that nativities taking place in a same sign have necessarily a similarity between them, yet they differ especially in sequence of the hereditary drawback, the Moon's motions and the rulership of the countries, etc., etc., although the nature of their maladies does not vary in type. Indeed those who are, for instance, of Saturn in Capricorn's type, may be affected of the following diseases which are of the same type: enteric fever, typhus, pulmonary catarrh, asthma, pulmonary emphysema, small pox, angina pectoris, syphilis, etc.

Hippocrates has instituted the doctrine of the crisis and criti-

---

[1]Mr. Alfred J. Pearce's *Almanac* for 1912.

Pathological Synthesis

cal days in the evolution of acute ailments. As long as medicine employed the simples and the physical agents, Nature's way of curing diseases was spared, but with the interference of chemistry, it lost its natural path, and so the sublime Hippocratic principle of crisis and critical days is looked at as a wreck of the ancient medicine. Nevertheless, it depends on the Moon's motion and action during the course of a Pyrexia. Indeed there is a direct connection between the fever and Moon's movements through the zodiac. So the fever is sometimes aggravated, sometimes mitigated and sometimes destroyed during the lunation, hence the occurrence of crisis and of critical days, the former being Nature's effort to get rid of the fever and the latter noticing the time in which the crisis may take place. Hippocrates said: "The lunar month has such especial power over our bodies, that not only birth but diseases, death, or recovery have a kind of dependence on such revolutions."[2]

Thus a continuous fever depends on the Moon's course through the zodiacal signs. But as she stays sometimes two days and sometimes three days in one of the zodiacal signs and pursues her course from sign to sign, a fever which began when the Moon was, for instance, in a X sign will cease to be judged when she comes to a sign whose elementary qualities oppose those of the Moon's quarter at her ingress into this sign. The Moon presents the following elementary qualities according to the quarters:

New Moon	Hot and moist
First Quarter	Hot and dry
Full Moon	Cold and dry
Last Quarter	Cold and moist

The zodiacal signs have the following elementary qualities:

Aries	Hot and dry
Taurus	Cold and dry

---

[2]Mr. A. J. Pearce's *Text-Book of Astrology*.

Gemini	Hot and moist
Cancer	Cold and moist
Leo	Hot and dry
Virgo	Cold and dry
Libra	Hot and moist
Scorpio	Cold and moist
Sagittarius	Hot and dry
Capricorn	Cold and dry
Aquarius	Hot and moist
Pisces	Cold and moist

The crisis is caused by one of the following eliminatory processes of humours: sweat, urine, vomiting, stools, haemorrhage, expectoration, eruptions, tumours. It may be advanced or delayed, complete, salutary, or lethal.

The critical days are the fourth, seventh, eleventh, fourteenth, twentieth, and twenty-sixth days from the day of decumbiture, which counts for one.

If the pyrexia is terminated in one of these days, it is said that the disease is judged. Besides, they permit to foretell what may happen in the course of the disease.

Using a chart set for April 17, 1912 at noon, it results that when a pyrexia takes place under a lunar sign it acquires the elementary qualities of the same, and that the disease may not come to termination (be judged) but when it reaches the lunar quarter of similar elementary qualities, ruling a sign of quite opposite elementary qualities.

So should the decumbiture take place on the second day of the lunar Aries (hot and dry), the disease acquires these elementary qualities, and may only be judged when it reaches the lunar first quarter: hot and dry in the sign Cancer, which is cold and moist. Thus the pyrexia will be judged the seventh day of the disease.

Let us continue. Should the fever take place on the second day of lunar Gemini (hot and moist), it will terminate on the twenty-sixth day of the disease when the Moon is new, hot and moist, and enters the sign Taurus, cold and dry, opposite to her elementary qualities, and so on.

The lunar course through the zodiac varies each month.

Thus, according to the elementary qualities of the lunar quarters and those of the signs, a pyrexia is either judged, mitigated, or aggravated in its symptoms, or pursues its course further on, beyond the twenty-sixth critical day. In this case, the disease changes of nature and passes to chronicity if death has not done its work.

The critical days doctrine is as true nowadays as it was at Hippocrates' time. But Hippocrates observed the disease's course and did not interfere with a disturbing medication, while our oftentimes unseasonable intervention troubles the disease's natural course and aggravates it.

Again the Hippocratic doctrine of crisis and critical days permits us to sustain the possibility to curtail the enteric or typhoid fever. This possibility was discussed. It is sure that when the pyrexia is judged on the eleventh day of its beginning (synocha) it is curtailed; if not, it is not curtailed. In both cases the fever is a typhoid one.

As to the prognostication of a pyrexia, it necessarily depends on the heavenly bodies geocentrically interfering in the course of the disease, as well as on the Moon's motions through the signs.

The planets may be classified in two classes: physiological and pathological.

The physiologicals are:
1. The Sun
2. The Moon and Venus
3. Mercury

and bring their action:

The Sun on the hematopoiesis.

The Moon and Venus on the chylopoiesis, and Mercury on both, as this latter borrows its influence of each of the two signs Virgo and Gemini of which it is the ruler, and which preside— Virgo to the chylopoiesis and Gemini to the haematopoiesis— dealing with all physiological and pathological processes.

The pathological planets are Mars, Jupiter, and Saturn, of which Mars and Jupiter preside to the haematopoiesis and Saturn to the chylopoiesis.

And it is of the human organism as it is of the plants, whose diverse parts differ in odor, taste, and propriety, in spite of the unity of the sap. The reason is that the macrocosm which presides over the formation of the different parts of the plant or the animal body (paracelsus) communicates to them these peculiarities according to the retrogressive metamorphosis of the cells.

Two properties, however, rule the matter: acidity and alkalinity, partaking of the organismic operations. If they are in due proportions in the body, a healthy state results, but as a standard healthy state is rather an exception, and thus, one of these two properties more or less prevails over the other.

I stated that the elementary qualities dry and Moist of the signs, are positive and negative in rotation, and as to the human body, the signs presiding over its right side are positive, head inclusive, and those occupying its left are negative, the feet inclusive.

The same will be considered in regard to the inward organs according as they are at the right (positive) or the left (negative) of the median line, and above (positive) and under (negative) the midriff (diaphragm).

Physiologically, the positive signs are alkaline and electro-positive; and the negative, acid and electro-negative.

So the qualities positive, or alkaline, and negative, or acid, design the taint on which evolves the diathesis or constitutional morbidity.

The sign ruling the country or the place of a nativity indicates the nature of the individual environment and typifies its hereditary tendencies. So whether it is a positive sign, it betrays, for the native, an electro-positive environment, and whether negative, an electro-negative environment.

This, also, is a necessary factor of the theme, and as extols Hippocrates, the natal country is often an important curative agent in many long diseases.

I will say that the division of the planets into positive and negative, acquiring a different meaning according to their nature, is a happy solution to the many psychological and biological problems hitherto remained unsolved; but I will add that, whether this distinction is true in regard to the male, positive by nature, the reverse would be true for a female, negative by nature. So a man whose solar sign is, for instance, Pisces, negative, there would be a Jupiterian negative, i.e., of a contrary potentiality to his own which is positive. A woman having the same nativity will be yet a Jupiterian negative, but of a similar potentiality to her own, which is negative. With the male Jupiter, ruler of Pisces, may be evil; with the female, good. Thus it would be unnecessary to deal with the Sun for a male, and the Moon for a female, in the meaning of a map, as their action as well as the planetary qualities depend on the signs.

For discovering the real meaning of life and its essential being, our researches would be fruitless if we did not try to discover it in ourselves, and that must be so because living matter does not indulge in analysis. Notwithstanding, life is certainly the effect of the action of a cause coming out of a living power, as nothing can grow of nothing. And as so, it must be an attribute of force and movement governing all the Universe, the matter and what we mean by it being but a property of them. So all links in Nature come out of the same evolving principle, all join together, and when the ovum becomes a man and the semen a flower, the laws that preside at these transmutations are always the same.

It is often spoken of as the soul of the world. This soul does not pertain to the Earth alone, but to the whole Universe of which our planet partakes. It is this universal soul that links the heavenly bodies constituting the macrocosm to the supreme being of the Earth, the man constituting the microcosm, and gives its potential of vitality to the cell.

"The notion of the continuity," says Mr. S. Meunier in his *Harmonies de revolution ierreslre*, "of the geological phenomena, and their persistency at our times in always the same way, is completed by the discovery in the Earth's structure of true anatomical apparatus, which bring us to the past's vitalistic intuitions, and to the constitution of a majestical and intensive state of life, to which the earthly mass obeys, resembling in a troubling matter a gigantic organism."

Indeed, compared to the Earth's structure, the human organism presents striking analogies. Thus the predominance of liquids on the solids; the inner perpetual movement keeping up the circulatory activity of the vital fluids; the duplicity of these fluids; first, the sea water, rich in vitality, and the arterial blood; second, the river water, the terrestrial water, poor of vitality, and the venous blood; the inner heat; the dew and the sweat; the rocks and the osseous frame; etc. Besides, either of our functions has its type, its identity in the intrinsical conformation of the Earth; and here and there life and death are operating in the same manner, i.e., through hot and cold, the inner cooling of the Earth being the way by which it would extinguish in an X period of time.

Pursuing further their study, we find that as matter is a propriety of Nature's forces, so the organic lesions, growths, tumours, etc., are the humoural manifestations of the body's direct psychical forces, or of indirect astro-meteoric, atmospheric, dynamic action on the humours. This explains the influence on the organism of colours, minerals, and all medicinal substances.

Pathological Synthesis

Chapter IX

Therapeutical Synthesis

Here's flowers for you,
Not Lavender; Mint; Savory; Marjoram
The Marigold that goes to bed with the Sun.
And with him rises, weeping; these are the flowers
Of Middle Summer, and I think they are
To men of middle age.—Shakespeare

The rule used in medicine," says Stahl, "to deal with diseases through remedies contrary or opposite to the effects they produce is entirely false and absurd. I am, on the contrary, convinced that they give up to the agents which cause a similar affection. And Paracelsus says, 'Nature rejoices with things of her nature, and of two different seeds no generations may come out; or it will be monstrous.'"

In alchemical operations, inferior or imperfect metals are transmuted into superior or perfect metals. They may follow the order hereafter: lead, Saturn; tin, Jupiter; iron, Mars; silver, Moon; copper, Venus; mercury, Mercury; and gold, Sun.

These diverse metals constitute the seven therapeutical pioneers for the treatment of diseases.

Besides, the law of signature (*ars signata*) served the ancients in their recognizing and classifying the therapeutical agents appropriated to the organs and diseases. So the nut which presents the form and the circumvolutions of the brain is a cephalic; the nutmeg, which resembles the cerebral substance, is a cephalic; the coffee seed whose two lobes present the form of the two cerebral lobes and that of the heart muscle is a cephalic and cardiac; the French-bean which resembles the kidneys (hence its appellation of kidney bean) is a renal and consequently an utmost cardiac; the Saw Palmetto *(sabal serrulata)* is a prostatic and acts on the ovaries and on the kidneys; the bitterness of the poison nut (*nux vomica*) designates it in bile affections, so it is not properly a hepatic; the platane, which sheds its bark annually, is, according to Dr. J. H. Clarke in *Dictionary of Materia Medica*, advantageously used in skin diseases.

"In Nature," says Paracelsus, "nothing is dead, and all that there is considered as material has a hidden soul in itself. . . . And so long as Man remained in Nature's state, he could get out the signatures of things, their virtues and properties, but in proportion as his spirit was subdued to the illusory appearances, he lost this power."

This law of signatures is the law by which we understand the universal language of Nature, which at first seems mysterious; but as soon as we face things and beings as they present themselves in their simplicity, it becomes clear and intelligible. Effectually, all that we call form in Nature's three kingdoms constitutes their signature, and the examination and observation of the form of the cranium, eyes, nose, ears, mouth, thorax, abdomen, the hands, the exterior form of the plants, the nature of their juices, textures, etc., etc., betray physiological, pathological, and therapeutical facts which result from the astral influences.

Although these signatures of things escape our investigation and scrutiny, yet we possess their astral correspondences such as are betrayed through tradition. I will resume them in the following pages, adding to them in the same time their chemical and therapeutical affinities. They will be classed in seven groups according to the seven heavenly bodies ruling them, as Uranus and Neptune were unknown to the ancients, so more so the action of these latter may be resumed in Saturn's.

Physiological Planets

Sun Group (ruler of Leo)

General action:
1. Stimulant
2. Tonic
3. Preservative

Physiological action:
1. Cerebro-spinal nervous system
2. Circulatory system
3. Tonicity, vital force

Chemical affinities:
Gold; equivalence 196
Platinum; equivalence 195
Iridium; equivalence 192.7

Therapeutical affinities:
Chamomilla, with its analogous remedies

And among the plants:
Angelica arehangelica: angelica; masterwort
Anethum nobilis: chamomille
Calendula officinalis: marigold
Citrus lemonum: lemon
Crocus sativus: saffron (the true)
Erythroea centaurium: centaury (small)
Euphrasia officinalis: eyebright
Helianthus annuus: sunflower
Hypericum perforatum: Saint John's wort

Juglans regia: walnut
Juniperus vulgaris: juniper
Laurus nobilis: laurel, bay tree
Mentha piperita: peppermint
Olea europea: olive tree
Pyrethrum parthenium: chamomille (wild)
Rosmarinus officinale: rosemary
Viscum album: mistletoe
Vitis vinifera: vine

Elementary qualities: hot and dry

Diathesis: cardiac

Mercury Group (ruler of Gemini and Virgo)

General action:
1. Nervine
2. Periodic

Physiological action:
1. Gastro-abdominal innervation through the solar plexus
2. Pulmonary innervation through the brachial plexus, and pulmonary haematosis
3. Nervous influx and periodicity

Chemical affinities:
Mercury; equivalence 200
Osmium; equivalence 192.2

Therapeutical affinities:
Bryonia alba and *nux vomica*, with analogous remedies

And among the plants:
Anethum foeniculum: fennel
Apium graveolens: celery (wild)
Apium petroselinum: parsley
Avena sativa: oat
Carum carvi: caraway

Therapeutical Synthesis

Daucus sylvestris: carrot (wild)
Clycyrhiza glabra: liquorice
Inula helenium: elecampane, elfwort
Lavandula spica: lavender of our gardens
Marrubium vulgare: horehound (white)
Melissa calaminta: balm or melissa
Origanum vulgare: marjoram (common)
Parietaria officinalis: pellitory
Pimpinella anisum: anise, aniseed
Saturea hortensis: savory

Elementary qualities: cold and dry

Diathesis: cranian

Venus Group (ruler of Taurus and Libra)

General action:
1. Fermentation (nutrition)
2. Proliferation

Physiological action:
1. Humoural secretions
2. Renal system
3. Glandular system

Chemical affinities:
Copper; equivalence 63
Zinc; equivalence 65

Therapeutical affinities:
Belladonna, *rhus loxicodendron*, with analogous remedies

And among the plants:
Achillea millefolium: yarrow, milfoil
Althaea officinalis: marshmallow
Aretium lappa: burrdock
Asparagus offlcinalis: asparagus
Bellis perennis: daisy

Fumaria offlcinalis: fumitory
Hibiscus eseulentus: okro, gombo pods
Malva sylvestris: mallow (common)
Nepeta glechoma: ivy (ground), alehoof
Phaseolus vulgaris: kidney bean
Plantago major: plantain (greater)
Potentilla anserina: sliverweed
Sambucus nigra: elder
Sanicula officinarum: selfheal
Saponaria officinalis: soapwort
Solidago virga aurea: golden rod

Elementary qualities: cold and moist

Diathesis: renal

Moon Group (ruler of Cancer)

General action:
   1. Zymotic
   2. Periodic (intermittence)

Physiological action:
   1. Sympathetic nervous system
   2. Mycrozymasis
   3. Zymotic periodicity

Chemical affinities:
   Silver; equivalence 108
   Palladium; equivalence 106.6

Therapeutical affinities:
   Ipeca, with its analogous remedies

And among the plants:
   Acorus calamus: flag (sweet)
   Cucurbita pepo: pumkin
   Lactuca sativa: lettuce
   Lemna minor: duck weed

Lilium candidum: lilly (meadow)
Lonicera caprifolium: woodbine, honeysuckle
Lunaria annua: moonwort
Mercurialis annua: Mercury weed
Nuphar lutea: water lily (yellow)
Portulaca oleracea: purslane
Sedum acre: betony stone-crop
Sedum telephium: livelong
Sisymbrium nasturtium: watercress

Elementary qualities: cold and moist, and according to quarters:
New Moon is hot and moist, and acts on the blood.
First Quarter is hot and dry, and acts on the bile.
Full Moon is cold and dry, and acts on the innervation.
Last Quarter is cold and moist, and acts on the lymph.

Diathesis: cranio-abdominal

Pathological Planets

Mars Group (ruler of Aries and Scorpio)

General action:
Sthenia

Pathological action:
1. Cerebro-spinal and sympathetic nervous system
2. Ductless glands, genito-urinary and renal systems
3. Vaso-dilatation
4. Inflammation

Chemical affinities:
Iron; equivalence 56
Manganese; equivalence 55
Nickel; equivalence 58.8
Coball; equivalence 58

Therapeutical affinities:
Aconitum napellus, pulsatilla, with analogous remedies

And among the plants:

Aloes socotrina: aloes
Artemisea absinthium: wormwood (common)
Arum maculatum: cooko pint
Bellis perennis: English daisy
Berberis vatgaris: Oregon grappe
Capsicum annuum: cayenne pepper
Carduus marianus: lady's thistle
Eupatorium aromaticum: white snake root
Gentiana latea: yellow gentian
Geranium maculatum: wild cranesbill
Gratiola ojicinalis: hedge hyssop
Hamamelis virginica: witch hazel
Humulus lupulus: hope
Juniperus sabina: savin
Myrica cerifera: wax myrtle, bayberry
Nicotiana rustica: tobacco
Ranunculas sceleratus: marsh crowfoot
Rheum palmatum: rhubarb
Rubia tinctorum: madder
Sabatia angularis: American centaury
Senna officinalis (cassia obovata): Alexandrian senna
Urtica urens: small stinging nettle

Elementary qualities: hot and dry

Diathesis: hepatic

Jupiter Group (ruler of Sagittarius and Pisces)

General action:
Perversion of the vital stimulus

Pathologioal action:
1. Muscular and fibro-ligamentous systems affecting the pulmonary parenchyma, the cardiac muscle, the gastro-intestinal tunics, and the vesical muscle (bladder)

2. Dyscrasia
3. Infection, toxemia

Chemical affinities:
    Tin; equivalence 118
    Antimony; equivalence 120
    Uranium; equivalence 120

Therapeutical affinities:
    Mercurius
    Veratrum album, with their analogous remedies

And among the plants:
    Agave americana: American aloe
    Agrimonia eupatoria: agrimony
    Borrago officinalis: borage
    Cichorium intibus: wild succory
    Cinnamomum (laurus): cinnamon
    Hyssopus officinale: hyssop
    Lichen istanditus: Iceland moss
    Lycopersicum esculentum: tomato, love apple
    Potentilla tormentilla: tormentil
    Rosa gallica: red rose
    Salvia officinalis: sage
    Scandix cerefolium: chervil
    Sempervivum tectorum: house leek
    Slicta pulmonaria: lung wort
    Taraxacum dens leonis: dandelion

Elementary qualities: hot and moist

Diathesis: thoracic

Saturn Group (ruler of Capricorn and Aquarius)

General action:
    1. Asthenia
    2. Stenosis

Pathological action:
1. Peripheral nerves
2. Cutaneous, mucous, and osseous systems
3. Connective tissue
4. Vaso-constriction
5. Degeneration of tissues

Chemical affinities:
Lead; equivalence 207
Bismuth; equivalence 208

Therapeutical affinities:
Aracaicum album
Sulphur, with their analogous remedies

And among the plants:
Aconitum lycoctonum: wolfsbane
Apocynum cannabinum: Indian hemp
Ceanothus americanus: New Jersey tea, red root
Hedera helix: common ivy
Hordeum bexasticon: barley
Polygonum hydropiper (persicaria urens): water pepper
Polypodium vulgare: rock polypod
Populus tremuluides: aspen poplar
Prunns spinosa: blackthorn
Quercus robur: English oak
Symphitum officinale: boneset
Verbascum thapsus: great mullein

Elementary qualities: cold and dry

Diathesis: splenic

Chapter X

The Practice

Prove all things; hold fast that which is good—Bible

The following pages constitute the keystone of what I exposed in the preceding chapters. Indeed, it would be useless to heap up materials without being able to use them to a practical purpose. I am aware of the difficulties inherent to the matter, but I will do my best to come to a satisfactory result, because what is missed more in astral medicine is not the materials but their resuming in a body for their possible application in practice.

One of the great laws of Nature is the division of all things and beings into two essential fundamental classes made up of positive and negative elements. These elements are, visibly or not, at the bottom of the whole of Nature's operations. The formation of new cells, that of embryo, the atmospheric, cosmic and telluric changes, etc., depend thereupon. The celebrated Brown based his medical doctrine on similar principles and his division of diseases into two classes: the sthenic and the asthenic, and this is but an adaptation of the positive and negative elements in medicine. It is true that prior to Brown the chemical physicians had asserted that disease was caused by an alkaline or acid humour. (Van Helmont, Ettmuller, etc.) Nevertheless, sthenic or asthenic, alkaline or acid, express but one and the same thing, as they are but the properties of the positive and negative elements, and result therefrom. The sole misconception of the iatro-chemists was to look at the disease as an entity by itself, when it depends on the individual himself. It is certain that two individuals, one alkaline and the other acid, may suffer from an identical nosological entity. But in both cases, it necessitates a different treatment in accordance with the individual drawback. That is the reason why a similar pathological treatment succeeds in one circumstance, and strands in some others. Besides, during an epidemic some persons easily catch the disease, while others are left immune. This is surely due to the morbid genus which attacks those whose vitality is below par.

"Part of the ideas here outlined are not new, for away hack in Hahnemann's day, we find," says Dr. Duncan in *Children, Acid and Alkaline*, "that he recognized the fact that the tendency to acidity was constant and abnormal."

This tendency easily is discovered through the signs ruling the conception point and the birth time. So it does not, all asserted, depend upon nourishment and care.

Now for establishing a therapeutical rule, let us observe a heliocentric map discussed in chapter VII.

The individual physiological formula resumed there is as follows:

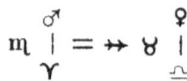

$$\mathfrak{m} \overset{\mathstrut\text{♂}}{\underset{\text{♈}}{|}} = \twoheadrightarrow \text{♉} \overset{\mathstrut\text{♀}}{\underset{\text{♎}}{|}}$$

That is to say, the individual physiological standard Scorpio Mars is Martian Mars negative Scorpio because the solar sign Scorpio is negative, predisposing the native to a humoural trouble Venus, in relation to the kidneys Libra, localizing in the throat and the naso-pharynx Taurus, and affecting the muscular system, then the heart, the gastro-intestinal tunics and the bladder Sagittarius.

As to the individual pathological formulae, they are resumed as hereafter, *vide* PAGES 92 AND 93:

First step:

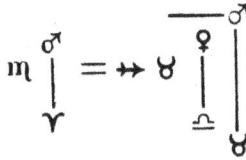

Second step:

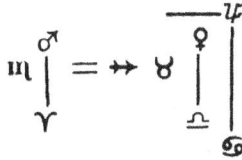

Third step:

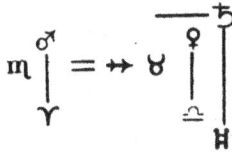

Thus the individual physiological standard gives way:

I. To a sthenic Mars nervous, Aries and Scorpio, humoural Venus disease of the throat and naso-pharynx with the above characteristics.

2. To an acquired toxaemic trouble Jupiter through the digestive organs Cancer.

3. To an acquired denutritive trouble Saturn affecting the respiratory organs and the pulmonary haematosis Gemini.

The reading of the formulae is made from the right to the left as in Arabian alphabet.

Now what would be the constitutional treatment?

It necessarily results from the physiological and pathological standards.

Indeed, I observe that only Taurus is common to both; that is to say it prevails especially in the subject's organic predispositions and morbidities, and that the remedies called for must have action on the organic systems betrayed by the signs, and be of the planetary groups of the heavenly bodies presiding to them in exponent.

Now let us see what is the sphere of action of the remedies needed in our case, and which remedies will agree with the native's predispositions and morbidities.

Mars is the pathological exponent of the formula partaking of the constitutional sign Taurus (by birth), so it marks the group of Martian remedies which will prevail in the treatment, and have action on the throat, the neck, the submaxillary glands and the naso-pharynx Taurus. Again, Mars ruling Scorpio and Aries, and Scorpio being the native's solar sign, they will further have action the ductless glands (hence the pituitary gland), the intestinal plexuses, the coecum, the large intestine, the rectum, and the genito-urinary organs, and act upon the nervous centers (the brain, the medulla, and the solar plexus) Aries. Besides, the Martian remedies will partake of the Venusian (Venus exponent) group's remedies which will be renal Libra, and have action on the throat, etc., Taurus. And both the Martian and Venusian remedies will oppose the muscular, cardiac, abdominal and vesical stenosis Sagittarius.

This constitutional drawback may predispose the native to a toxaemic disease Jupiter of the gastric organs Cancer affecting the muscular system, then the heart, the gastro-intestinal tunics and the bladder Sagittarius, and the fibro-ligamentous system and the feet Pisces. So the remedies will be of the Jupiterian group Jupiter and have action on the above organic systems Sagittarius and Pisces. Still these remedies will partake of the qualities of Mars and Venus remedies.

Now, in consequence of Jupiter's disease, may be unfolded a tedious complaint Saturn grafted on the individual physiological standard Scorpio Mars, giving way to a trouble of the respiratory organs and the pulmonary haematosis Gemini in their connection with the peripheral nerves and circulation Capricorn and the sanguineous system Aquarius. So the remedies called for will be of the Saturnian group and have action on the pulmonary parenchyma Gemini, the peripheral nerves and circulation Capricorn and the blood (lack of red corpuscles) Aquarius. Again, the Saturnian group's remedies will partake of the qualities of Mars, Jupiter, and Venus remedies.

It is to be observed that Mars and Saturn, with their ruling signs, especially characterize any morbid evolution, as this latter manifests through the nervous cell's irritation, or atony, and the medical agent or agents resulting from, will take part in a combination of Mars and Saturn remedies. So Rademacher's acetate of iron[1] would be a universal remedy as it is composed of sulphate of iron Mars and acetate of lead Saturn, i.e., through the precipitation of Saturn by Mars. It implicates "a copious alkaline urine or less copious and acid urine," and suits as well to acute (febrile) and chronic ailments; but its action must be completed by an organismic remedy, be it hepatic, splenic or renal[2]. Unhappily this preparation is an unsteady one, and must be freshly prepared and used.

---

[1] Rademacher's *Universal and Organ Remedies.*
[2] These remedies are greater celandine, poison nut, lady's thistle, saffron, quassia, vegetable charcoal, squill, acorns of English oak, juniper berries, yellow amber, hemlock *(conium maculatum)*, galeopsis, golden rod, cochineal, New Jersey tea *(ceanothus americanus)*.

Dr. Schussler's *ferrum phosphoricum* Mars may be a good substitute to it, but it should be taken in rotation with *kali phosphoricum*, a Saturnian remedy.

Paracelsus and Hahnemann have righteously inveighed against polypharmacy in which reigned the utmost incoherence.

However, all in Nature is complex, and a remedy because it is dispensed alone does not exclude the complexity. Nevertheless, this is far from mixing together, in a phial, incongruous or heterogenous substances. The practitioner must know to take advantage of a medication, and combine it according to circumstances. Thus the water is but a combination of O and H; yet it would be insufficient to put in presence these elements for obtaining water. For this purpose, it would be necessary to establish their right proportions, and afterwards pass them through an electric discharge. Notwithstanding neither O nor H alone can form water, and unfold its properties.

Now let us consider the same nativity at the solar-lunar standpoint. The chart discussed in chapter VII will serve our purpose.

First: tonality, Mars and Mercury in, respectively, Scorpio and Cancer, and Aries; modalities, Moon in Taurus, and Libra.

That is to say the remedies will be of Martian and Mercurian groups tonality and have action on the ductless glands (the pituitary gland inclusive), the intestinal plexuses, the coecum , the large intestine, the rectum and the genito-urinary organs Scorpio, further on the digestive system Cancer, and as to the modalities, on the throat, neck, and submaxillary glands, the naso-pharynx Taurus and the renal secretory system.

Second, zones six, seven, and eight vide MAP PAGE 98, which are under the esoteric planetary action Saturn, Jupiter, and Mars and mark the action of the remedies through Aries, Taurus, and Gemini, i.e., the organic systems betrayed by these signs with regard to Virgo and Scorpio.

Third, the esoteric planets Sun, Moon, Mercury's zones, and Sagittarius, Pisces, and Aquarius in regard to Taurus, Leo, and Cancer.

Thus the two systems lead to the same result with the difference that the solar-lunar system is more complex than the heliocentric. It is obvious that for whoever is aware of the humoural pathogeny, the reflex action of the nervous ganglia and plexuses on the organic systems, and the pathogenesis of the remedies, the heliocentric system joins, to a scientific basis in accordance with the universal laws governing the celestial bodies, the Earth, and man, a simplicity and an accuracy which are subsidiary to truth.

So the remedies intervening in the constitutional treatment of the native, will be, as I have stated in the generalities, dispensed through the law of similars and the dietetic measures suiting him, will be prescribed according to the law of contraries.

It is to be observed that the nervous centers of the viscera constitute a great nervous unity; they are between them fastened through the nerve cords, influenced reciprocally in their functions, and influence themselves for unfolding the disease. Thus any pathological affection of an abdominal viscera may be the cause of a disease of a thoracic viscera as they depend one on the other.

Yet the sympathetic nervous system which presides over the organic life in its functions is continually influenced by the medulla and cerebral nervous cells which put it in relation with the cerebro-spinal nervous system. So each viscera in function impresses the medulla and the brain, and invertedly the brain and medulla react on the visceral functions, forming between them a nervous unity which secures the organismic unity, leading, in its turn, to the pathological one, which necessarily results from the astral unity. Indeed let us suppose a nativity taking place in Gemini. Besides, the native's Mercury is in Sagittarius, Venus in Taurus, Uranus in Sagittarius, Moon in Libra, Mars in Scorpio, Jupiter in Pisces, and Saturn in Cancer. Hence the formula hereafter:

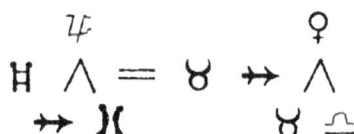

$$\begin{array}{ccccc} & ♃ & & & ♀ \\ ♅ & \wedge & = & ♉ & ⇀ & \wedge \\ & ⇀ &)(& & ♉ & ♎ \end{array}$$

Thus the native is threatened by birth of a toxaemic ailment Jupiter affecting the muscles of the thighs Sagittarius and of the feet Pisces through the pulmonary haematosis Gemini (polymyelitis paralysis infantilis).

Hence, humoural trouble Venus by insufficient elimination of the secretion products Libra and the atony of the muscular system Sagittarius threatening the Eustachian tube Taurus (possible deafness).

The other pathological planets Mars and Saturn threaten: the first Scorpio, and the second Cancer.

That is to say, Mars threatens: Scorpio, and its homological organic system Taurus, i.e., the naso-pharynx Scorpio through the eustachian tube Taurus (nervous irritative dizziness).

And Saturn threatens: Cancer and its homological organic system Capricorn, i.e., the digestive organs Cancer through the peripheral nerves and circulation Capricorn (atony of the digestive organs, hence obstinate costiveness).

It is to be observed the near similarity existing between the above formula and that shown in the previous illustration in this chapter as to the second part of the equations. In the latter Sagittarius occupies the first rank, and in the first Taurus occupies this place. Both then evolve nearly similarly, but the latter on Scorpio Mars Aries and the first on Gemini Jupiter Sagittarius Pisces. So they differ essentially between ween themselves and produce a different type and different morbid manifestations.

An important point to be noted is the role of the nervous cell and blood in living bodies. Indeed, the blood, which has charge of the nutrition (fuel) of the tissues, and the nervous cell,which rules the blood's circulation and innervation (its distribution to the tissues) are the only factors of the organism, as well as those of the pathological condition. So long as health is maintained the nervous cell accomplishes its functions without noticing its existence, but as soon as its action becomes sensible, a pathological process is extant. This sensibility of the nervous cell is what constitutes its irritation which affects the blood.

Thus the ovum is formed of the nervous cell (positive) and the blood (negative).

The nervous cell is the attribute of the vital force, and the blood constitutes the matter of which is formed the cell. So all in Nature is the result of force (positive) and matter (negative), since, as Buchner righteously asserts, there is no force without matter, and no matter without force.

In its turn, the blood gives way to the bile (a combustion product eliminated from the economy) and to the splenic humour (another combustion product storaged in the economy), and to an excess of the white corpuscles, hence the temperaments as we have seen elsewhere.

In conclusion, the therapeutical agents will, first, depend on the nervous cell; second, on the blood, and incidentally, on the bile and the splenic humour, as regulators of these latter.

As to the germs (microbes), surely they accompany the morbid excreta as they are but produced through the diseased excretory matters exposed to the air and ambiency (decomposition) and they may not be formed in closed cavities of the economy. (Dr. Middendorp) So the germ or microbe is but an effect of a hidden cause, and is not only destroyed by the solar rays, but yet for its possible development it necessitates a favorable milieu, and the troubles which are produced by its intravenous injection in the circulation, constitute but a false pathological process due to a heterogenous and virulent matter introduced in the economy.

The organic lesion, too, is a sequel of the nervous cell's irritation. Indeed, when one of the links of the nervous chain is suffering, it does not suffer alone, all the nervous chain of which it is a link resents bye and by this irritation, thus affecting the whole nervous frame.

So the breach of the nervous chain may take place through the irritation of some center, as the brain, the medulla, or the plexus of a viscera. When it is through the brain, headache, vertigo, and insomnia will result first; afterwards the cerebral irritation will drag the medullar irritation, hence neuralgias, sensory organic troubles, and ultimately it may attain a visceral plexus, i.e., the solar plexus or the cardiac plexus, or the pulmonary plexus and give way to dyspepsia, angina pectoris, or palpitations, or a pulmonary affection as bronchitis, pleuritis, etc., and the symptoms resulting from will be invertedly produced whether the primary affection's nervous center is that of a viscera. Nevertheless, this morbidly affected center's progression may take place quickly or slowly, and give way meanwhile, in semblance, to multiple and several diseases which have but one origin: the nervous center. The recovery of the health is possible but when the equilibrium of the whole nervous centers is obtained, and the nervous unity is reconstituted. (Dr. Leven)

Thus, diseases nosologically classified present but objective symptoms, and do not mean a morbid independent entity by themselves.

As to the acute and epidemic diseases, they depend also on the nervous unity.

Chapter XI

The Therapeutics of Chronic Ailments

Nature always works simply—Roger Bacon

There are three proceedings which serve to establish the sphere of action of a remedy. They are:

1. Through the law of signature, uncertain nowadays.

2. Through the clinical principles, varying according to the medical theories of the moment.

3. Through its being tested on a healthy man, the only true, because it is in accordance with Nature's law: *similia similibus*.

So this latter perfectly responds to all therapeutical needs.

A second great law of Nature is the polarity ruling things and beings.

Thus the therapeutical agents must be divided in two classes:
1. Electro-positive or alkaline
2. Electro-negative or acid

Yet they do not enjoy these qualities neither in the same

manner nor proportions. Hence a gradation to establish in their sphere of action.

The classification of the remedies, proved on the healthy, constitutes the homeopathic system. But what is missing to them is their division according to the polarity subsidiary to each one.

Dr. C. von Boenninghausen, in order to accomplish this end, established the drug affinity on the sides of the body, and in numerous cases where the lack of decisive symptoms rendered the selection of the proper remedy doubtful, it was mostly helpful.

The ancients too were aware of this law of polarity (alkaline or acid) of the drugs, as they classed them in hot and dry, hot and moist, cold and dry, cold and moist, at the first, second, third, and fourth degree. This was a great step made toward the truth. But the principle of *contraria contrariis* hindered to take advantage of it, and these distinctions are now obsolete. Nevertheless, it would be possible to establish them on a new account. The following proceeding will give us a satisfactory result. It is true, it misses scientific accuracy, but it will be with it as it is with the organoleptic examination of the urines; this latter misses also of a scientific accuracy, yet it is invaluable for the practitioner in the diagnosis and prognosis of diseases.

This proceeding will consist in the first sight effects produced by some acid-tests on the different substances of the three kingdoms of Nature.

The acid-tests which will serve our purpose are:
1. Nitric acid
2. Murialic acid
3. Sulphuric acid

The effects, the mixing or contact of one of these acids with a substance may produce, are the following:
1. A bubbling
2. An elevation or rise

3. A cracking
4. An effervescence
5. An exhalation

The effect produced may be greater, smaller, or null.

When it is null, it marks that the basic elements of the substances are rather acid; when it is smaller, it denotes that they are somewhat alkaline; and when it is greater, it betrays their greatest degrees of alkalinity.

In a general way, vegetables produce little effect, and animal products more.

Thus we presume that vegetables contain a small quantity of volatile or lixivial alkaline salt varying with the different parts of the vegetable, and this quantity is sometimes so small that it needs to be distinguished through a microscope or magnifying glass.

For instance, *colocynth* produces a smaller effect than any other vegetable hardly cathartic. So its cathartic action is due but to an acid principle, and drastic action may be amended with some alkaline substance.

The *spurge* (euphorbia corollata) with nitric acid produces a great effect, so is but an alkaline resin and cathartic. That is the reason why it relieves the irritation of the mucous surfaces and promotes their functional activity.

The *pips of pears* make with nitric acid a greater effect than with other vegetables. So they possess greatest medicinal virtues, although they have not been used in medicine. They may constitute a curative agent of value in nephritis and nephretic diseases.

The *lapis lazuli* with nitric acid produces a perceptible effect. Thus, its cathartic action is due to an alkaline principle; hence its usefulness in hypochondriasis which is entertained by an individual acid diathesis. So it is with iron.

Nevertheless, in this case as in all cases where the contraries are used, it is through their palliative action that the remedies amend the disease but do not cure it. The contraries simply allow Nature or a remedy used according to the similarity, to achieve the cure. The same happens with the dietetics, which are unable to cure a disease but serve at the most to alleviate its symptoms. Indeed, it would be a pity for a sick man to drudge with alimentary restrictions during his whole life.

Another of Nature's laws is that any chronic disease may not be cured by a sole remedy as there is no specific one unless the disease be functional. Oftentimes a unic remedy seems to be curative. But in similar cases we forget to consider the prior remedies used: allopathic or homeopathic. It is through their reaction together with the ultimate remedy's action that the cure is obtained. Indeed, in chronic ailments, just as the organism took time to get weak, it will take time to get strong, and a chronic disease is always a complex one.

It is only through the individual astral chart that we may arrive at its accurate treatment.

The points to be considered in this case are:
1. The pathological formula resulting from the individual chart of the ruling planets which mark the group of remedies.
2. The same for establishing the polarity of the remedies through the signs.
3. The individual constitution or temperament.
4. The season and its qualities, at the beginning of the treatment.

A simple way to denote the therapeutical agents from the astral data would be to classify and number the heavenly bodies:

Aries	Gemini	Leo	Libra	Sagittarius	Aquarius
1	3	5	7	9	11

are positive signs, and bring odd numbers, and

Taurus	Cancer	Virgo	Scorpio	Capricorn	Pisces
2	4	6	8	10	12

are negative signs, and bring even numbers.

The planets are not numbered because their role is not passive as it is with the signs, which they actuate and vibrate according to their potentialities.

☉	☿	♀	☽	♂	♃	♄
+	+-	-	-	+++	++	---

Now, here are twelve typical polychrest remedies corresponding to the twelve zodiacal signs,

+	1 -	♈ -	Aconitum napellus	+ or -
-	2 -	♉ -	Belladonna	+ or -
+	3 -	♊ -	Bryonia alba	+ or -
-	4 -	♋ -	Ipeca	+ or -
+	5 -	♌ -	Chamomilla	+ or -
-	6 -	♍ -	Nux vomica	+ or -
+	7 -	♎ -	Rhus toxicodendron	+ or -
-	8 -	♏ -	Pulsatilla	+ or -
+	9 -	♐ -	Mercurius	+ or -
-	10 -	♑ -	Sulphur	+ or -
+	11 -	♒ -	Arsenicum album	+ or -
-	12 -	♓ -	Veratrum album	+ or -

The Rosicrucian remedies were also twelve.

Let us proceed with an illustration: Mr. X. was born November 14, 1883 at 3:00 pm. His Sun occupies 22° Scorpio, decanate Cancer, and his Moon occupies 19° Taurus. These signs are negative, so he is vibrating negatively and the ailments to which he is subject are subsidiary to

Scorpio =   8
Cancer =   4
Taurus =   2
            14[1]
Less   12
             2

and 2 equals belladonna.

On the other hand, the native's physiological standard is as follows:

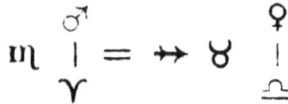

$$♏ \ | \ \overset{♂}{\underset{♈}{}} = \ ⇸ \ ♉ \ \overset{♀}{\underset{♎}{}} |$$

These signs vibrate as hereafter, Sagittarius excepted.

- Scorpio =   -8
+ Aries =   +1
+ Sagittarius = (9)
- Taurus =   -2
+ Libra =   +7   ___
                     +8   -10

namely: + 8 equal pulsatilla +
- 10 equals sulphur -, and Sagittarius = (9)
= mercurius will constitute an intercurrent remedy, since Sagittarius, not being innervated by any planet, is neutral.

Besides, the dominant ruling planets being first Mars and second Venus, the remedies will be of Martian-Venusian vibration, and have action on the muscular system, i.e., heart (muscle), gastro-abdominal tunics, and bladder (muscle), noticed by Sagittarius, neutral.

At this point, I observe that aconit, a Martian drug, and belladonna, a Venusian drug, act on the muscular system *(vide*

[1]When the total exceeds 12, deduct this and consider the remainder.

pathogenesis)[1]; so these remedies suit, and will partake of the treatment to which belladonna already pertains, so aconite alone must be added. Further, these remedies will supply to:
1. The individual temperament
2. The character of the season

If they do not, then we need to search for another analogous remedy. In our case, the temperament is nervous, and the season cold and wet leading up to the spring. Now, belladonna[2] especially responds to these characters so we need not search for another remedy.

It will be observed that where there is a pathological planet in the· physiological standard, it is this planet which gives to the formula its tonality. If there is any, then the ruling physiological planet of the first member of the equation will be the preponderating one. To sum up:

aconit + + + (Martian remedy)
and Pulsatilla +

combine together in the proportions of three parts of the former-and one part or the latter, and

belladonna -
and sulphur -

do it in one part of each, and these two groups of remedies in rotation constitute Mr. X.'s constitutional and fundamental treatment, with mercurius as intercurrent.

Now let us observe the Moon's monthly transit through the native's solar sign because in chronic ailments the remedies manifest their full action from this moment. This is the reason why drugs act more or less promptly with everybody. In special pathological cases, the signs, exclusively threatened by the pathological planets, will be considered and the fundamental treatment reinforced accordingly. Besides, in case of need, it is an

[1]Coperthwaite's *Materia Medica*.
[2]*Boenninghausen's Repertory* by H.C. Allen.

easy matter to get out similar and complementary drugs to the twelve polychrests of our scheme by means of Boenninghausen's or D. John H. Clarke's *Repertory*[1].

It is obvious that these rules apply to homeopathic remedies and posology, both of which are derived from Nature's great law of similars. So they are not connected with the official school, which depends on the dominant theories of the moment, and the empiricism!

The usual attenuations of the remedies are the 6X for vegetables, and the 12X for minerals and animal products. In special cases, they may go up from 30X to 200X.

---

[1] *Clinical Repertory*. Homeopathic Publishing Co., London. Also *Bird's Eye Repertory*.

Chapter XII

The Therapeutics of Acute Diseases

Omnia Vincit Veritas.

The acute diseases are dependent on the year's, season's and country's constitutions.

The year's constitution results from the planetary cycle and circles.

For instance, 1910's constitution is formed from Mars' cycle and the Sun's circle, i.e., from positive elements. So it was bilious.

As to the seasons, they have in a general way the following potentialities:

    Spring + i.e., Sanguine
    Summer + + i.e., Bilious
    Autumn - - i.e., Nervous
    Winter - i.e., Lymphatic

Nevertheless, these potentialities vary according to the planetary configurations of each season. So the spring 1910 celestial figure, through the physiological formula, gives way to the following equation:

$$ \Upsilon \overset{\text{♄}}{\underset{\text{♌ ♒}}{\wedge}} = \; \underline{\Omega} \quad \underline{\Omega} \quad \overset{\odot}{\underset{\text{♌}}{|}} $$

Where:

Saturn holds of Aquarius' nature, and the Sun holds of Leo's nature, these signs being exponents of which the esoteric Saturn and the Sun predominate.

That is to say, the spring of 1910, promoting the blood and the circulation, had a sanguineous constitution affecting the renal system Libra.

The summer of the same year results in the equation:

$$ \text{♋} \overset{\text{♄}}{\underset{\text{♌ ♒}}{\wedge}} = \; \text{♓} \; \text{♌} \; \overset{\text{♄}}{\underset{\text{♒}}{|}} $$

Saturn holds of Aquarius' nature. That is to say, the summer, through the heavenly configurations, acquired an asthenic sanguineous constitution affecting the fibro-ligamentous and synovial system Pisces.

Autumn 1910 results in the equation:

$$ \underline{\Omega} \overset{\text{♃}}{\underset{\text{♂ ♓}}{\wedge}} = \; \text{♌} \; \Upsilon \; \overset{\text{☿}}{\underset{\text{♅ ♍}}{\wedge}} $$

Jupiter holds of Pisces' nature and Mercury holds of Virgo's nature.

That is to say the autumn, through the heavenly configurations, acquired a sanguineous plethoric Jupiter nervous Mercury constitution, affecting the circulatory system Leo.

The winter map of the same year results in the equation:

$$\begin{array}{ccccc}
& ♃ & & & ☿ \\
♑ & \wedge & = & ♑ \;\; ♋ & \wedge \\
& ♂ \;\; ♓ & & & ♅ \;\; ♍
\end{array}$$

Jupiter holds of Pisces' nature, and Mercury holds of Virgo's nature. That is to say, the winter, through the heavenly configurations acquired a serous plethoric nervous constitution affecting the peripheral nerves and the cutis.

And the four seasons evolved on the bilious constitution, this latter being that of the year 1910.

As to the constitution of the countries and towns, it results from their ruling signs noticing that:

Aries, Leo, and Sagittarius are bilious.

Taurus, Virgo, and Capricorn are nervous.

Gemini, Libra, and Aquarius are sanguine.

Cancer, Scorpio, and Pisces are lymphatic.

So these data are of utmost usefulness in the cure of epidemic diseases, ague, and other acute ailments, and they will be of not less advantage in the cure of chronic complaints where the remedies being in accordance with the constitution of the year, season, and country, will operate more surely. That is what the ancients called the *genus epidemicus*.

Indeed, it is a nosological fact that besides the general ailments there are a certain number of special acute diseases that are peculiar to certain countries where they reign endemically. It is believed that sometimes they leave their original boundary and spread away epidemically, returning to their primarily localities after a short pilgrimage (Dr. Chapiel). It rather seems to me that they never do leave the limits of their original countries and when a similar ailment is observed elsewhere, it is because the telluric, cosmic, and astral conditions giving way to the endemic disease, have been established there: the same causes producing the same effects. Nevertheless, the disease in its new focus, changes of nature and is but transitory, because 1)it is of a different potentiality than that of the country where it is endemic, hence its epidemicity; and 2) the astral configurations giving way to its eclosion are not everlasting, hence its trasitoriness.

Now, for the cure to institute in an acute disease, let us proceed with an illustration. Mr. X, age 35, was taken ill with a fever on the 5th of March 1910. He lives in Paris, France.

So, he is an adult and of nervous temperament, 1910's constitution:

Cycle = Mars   = Bilious
Circle = Sun`   = Bilious

Season's constitution = winter = *serous plethoric nervous.*
Town = Virgo   = *Bilious-nervous*
Country = Leo   = *Bilious-nervous*

Thus the disease will be bilious-nervous (aconitum) of an abdominal origin (veratrum album) because of winter = serous-plethoric nervous, and the fever will be high, with muscular pains (over-fatigue) so the Moon on the 5th of March 1910 was in Sagittarius, a fiery sign affecting the muscular system. But it will be ephemeral because the Moon's Last Quarter = cold and moist in Sagittarius = hot and dry.

Should the disease have begun under another sign, it would have pursued its course for some days or farther.

Then it is necessary to take account of the Moon's action according to the lunar phases ruling the beginning and the course of the disease.

Here is a scheme of Moon's phases remedies:
New Moon—alumina, ammonium carb, caustieum, clematis, cuprum, mezereum, sabadilla, sepia, silicea
First Quarter—alumina, arnica, clematis, mezereum
Full Moon—alumina, calcarea carb, cyclamen, graphites, natrun carb, sabina, sepia, silicea, spongia, sulphur
Last Quarter—alumina, calcarea carb, dulcamara, graphites, silicea, thuya

Thus if an acute disease has begun during the New Moon and passes to the First Quarter, to Full Moon, the remedies of the former will prevail until the First Quarter, and then those of this latter until the Full Moon, and so on.

As to the selection of the remedies, it results from their pathogenetic action with regard to the symptoms of the disease and its cause.

It is observed that a remedy during months or a year, or at certain times, acts brightly and then suddenly ceases to do so. The reason of this is the moment's constitution, consequently of that of the disease. So long as it remains unaltered, the remedy acts; but as soon as it changes, the same remedy is useless. The qualities electro-positive (alkaline) and electro-negative (acid) of the ambiency do not apparently alter the symptoms of a disease, but yet the latter differs in its essence. So the ironical assertion in regard to a boasted remedy—"to make haste to use it when it cures"—contains a great therapeutical truth. It is also the reason why some forgotten remedies are from time to time desinterred and extolled. The maladies of special organs, as eyes and ears, are frequently independent of a general affection; they often depend on the introduction of a foreign or irritant body, dust or hardened cerumen, and consequently they need a local external treatment. Nevertheless, sometimes eyes may suffer (amblyopia, amaurosis, etc.) from a sympathetic affection caused by hyperacidity of the alimentary canal, in which case, says Rademacher, laxatives or anti-acids are the remedy, or it may be a reflex of a primary affection of some other organ, which organ must first be cured. The selection of the remedy for eye diseases changes with the time, one year requiring this remedy, another year that one.

"Nose affections, such as loss of smell, chronic choryza, ulceration," pursues Rademacher, "are often reflex symptoms of an abdominal affection, cure this, and the other will disappear too."

So since the great Siberian or Russian epidemic of La Grippe or influenza that ravaged Europe and America more than a quarter of a century ago, and which was so lethal, many small and endemic forms of the same followed. These latter were somewhat less murderous, yet malignant, and gave way to chronical toxoemic phenomena affecting the nervous system, hence a new morbid entity: neurasthenia, which is as proteiform as La Grippe, and whose localization, like that of the latter, is in the naso-pharynx, Virgo ruler Mars. So it is necessary not to confound this neurasthenia with brain fag, the general nervous weakness and the constitutional nervousness. Besides, the most troubling and tenacious symptom of neurasthenia is sleeplessness, or more accurately the awakening of the sick at 2:00 am, which marks a periodicity. So Galen was right in considering stubborn insomnia as a fever of an intermittent type and in advising to cure it accordingly.

Galen extolled the following cure:
    Poppy heads
    Lettuce seeds
    Violet flowers
    Myrtle leaves

Make a strong decoction. Wash with it the feet, the thighs, and the legs. Dry, rubbing softly at first, and harshly afterwards, with a flannel, a brush, or a rough linen, and then go to bed.

The country as a multiple center of peculiar astral and telluric influence plays a great role in the formation of the individual constitution and diseases. This is the reason why the American or exotic species of a plant suit better the natives of those countries than the European species of the same, and vice versa. Besides, each country has its flora, so that God put by the side of the disease, its remedy.

The house leek, a Jupiterian plant, crushed with flour of barley (Saturn) and olive oil (Sun) is heroic in curing ring worm, eczema and all inflammatory skin troubles, yet it may not be truly curative except with those who are born under a Jupiterian sign (Sagittarius or Pisces) and have Jupiter in Sagittarius or Pisces, and Saturn in Capricorn of Aquarius.

The seeds of the small stinging nettle, a Martian plant, boiled in wine (Sun) cure inflammatory affections of the lungs and pleura with those born in Aries or Scorpio, and have Mars in Gemini.

The conserve made with the seeds of purslain or honeysuckle, a lunar plant, constitutes the best cure for asthma for those whose birth sign is Cancer and have the Moon in Gemini.

The juice of aloe (Mars) mixed with vinegar (Saturn) forms a lotion which surely stops the falling of the hair with those born under a Martian sign having Saturn in Capricorn or Aquarius.

The juice of bananas drunk in three or four wineglassfuls a day would be very efficacious in tuberculosis, but this cure does not succeed but with those who are natives of the countries where the banana tree grows and are born under the sign of the banana's ruling planet; and so on with the plants.

Now what about the mineral kingdom?

Is is not the first component of all Nature's works? And, as so, a living matter? That is the reason why the alchemists spoke always of the fermentation (nutrition) of metals; but this process is as unseen and mysterious as that of the transmutation of the cell or ovum, and both escape our investigations, as does the essence of life. Notwithstanding, it is so, and the elixir of life, i.e., the philosopher's stone, depends on it. Belonging to the great whole, constituting the fundamental elements of the organic and inorganic matters, the minerals, classified according to the Mendelejeff's law in seven (ancient number of planets) or nine (modem division of planets), should rule all the therapeutical matters. Yet it is not through their chemical properties but through their psychical, vitalistic, dynamic virtues of which partakes anyone of the substances belonging to the three kingdoms, that we must consider the minerals. Have not the seven traditional planetary metals the following peculiar psychical characteristics?

Mars, iron, choleric
Sun, gold, personal
Moon, silver, timorous
Venus, copper, mutable
Mercury, mercury, agitated
Jupiter, tin, tempered
Saturn, lead, melancholic

Moreover, are not colours a property of living metals? Can we be indifferent to their influences on the mind? Is not red exciting; blue soothing ; orange stimulating; yellow relaxing; green restful; violet sedative as well as indigo?

It is evident that the seven colours of the spectrum ought to be also those of the planets. Still the astrological colours differ from them. Nevertheless, red seems to be Mars' colour, orange the Sun's colour, yellow the Moon's colour, blue Venus's colour; green Mercury's colour; indigo Jupiter's colour, and violet Saturn's colour.

Indeed, we observe: 1) that the red Mars and the violet Saturn are antagonistic, and so they must be, 2) that the red Mars and the green Mercury form the orange, i.e., the Sun's colour; 3) that the red Mars and the blue Venus give way to the purple, the Kabala's colour for Jupiter; 4) that the yellow Moon and the blue Venus form the green, Mercury's colour, and the symbol of this latter is but Venus surmounted of the Moon, i.e., Mercury, that the typical colours are the red Mars; the yellow Moon; the blue Venus.

Now, should a functional trouble come in (astral conflagration, consequently humoural conflagration), a pathological state is the result and may be either single or complex.

If it comes out through Mars, it would be by alteration of hepatic functions and give way to acute and sthenic diseases, hence Mars remedies and colour will be curative by sympathy; if it comes out through Jupiter, it would be by alteration of pulmonary and hepatic haematosis, and hence Jupiter remedies and colour will be curative; and if it is through Saturn, it would be through splenic functions and give way to chronic and asthenic diseases and Saturn remedies and colour will be curative.

Besides, as living matter, the minerals too will have their disease and die. "Certain metallic elements," says the Lancet, "have their sickness, but perhaps the tin plague is the most remarkable. If tin catches cold it will decay, it will lose its lustre, and finally crumble to a grey powder. The change is not a chemical one, for the grey powder is still tin, and it can be brought back by careful warming to its original healthy condition. Apparently, when the tin is very pure it is more susceptible to cold and consequent decay. In fact, it may be made proof against the disease by alloying it with other metals. The disease is a source of considerable annoyance and disappointment to the collectors of coins who possess valuable tin specimens in their cabinets. This curious toiling of tin may possibly have led to the use of the word tin as a term of reproach, as in such expressions as a tin-pot institution or a tin soldier, even tin buttons have been known to crumble in their way, and organ pipes made of tin have been found to decay after a severe winter. Tin rot, to keep up the analogy of disease, is even infectious, for decaying tin in contact with healthy lustrous, tin soon spoils it and reduces it to its own unhealthy stale. If tin is to be protected effectually against the ravages of cold, it should be kept above 18°C. The best remedy appears to be, however, to alloy it with another metal, notably lead. There are many mysterious things about the inanimate, and the illness of certain metallic elements forms one of them. The energetic colloidal form of platinum can be poisoned or rendered inactive by prussic acid or corrosive sublimate; or mercury gets sick in contact with other metals; glass gets fatigued under electric stress so that it will no longer transmit certain rays until it has had a few days rest; silver spits just as it changes from the molten to the solid state. In certain instances the illness referred to has been a serious drawback to the use of metals in industrial and domestic applications, but fortunately the disease usually yields to treatment based upon the diagnosis of the metallurgical chemist

Chapter XIII

The Hygiene

Joy, contentment and Repose.
Slam the door on the doctor's nose.—Old Saw[1]

Here are the seven hygienic laws of Hoffmann, the celebrated German physician of the 17th century:

1. Avoid all excesses.

2. Never bring sudden changes in your habits.

3. Keep calm your spirit and avoid sadness.

4. Choose a pure and tempered air.

5. In your foods, select those suiting your temperament, taste and habit.

6. Preserve an equilibrium between your nourishment and exercises.

7. Avoid physics, and I will add taking cold.

Moreover, in order that the alimentation may be easily assimilated and of profit, it is necessary:

---

[1]Dr. Schofield. *How to Keep Fit.* 1910. William Rider & Son, London.

1. That the solid foods coming out of the animal and vegetal kingdoms be eaten with pleasure and not with disgust, and reluctantly.

2. That they must be thoroughly masticated, which is obtained through only good teeth.

3. That the alimentary bolus must abide in the intestines.

4. That the drinks (wine, beer, cider) must be of a good quality and age.

5. That the exercises must he proportioned to the quantity of food, and according to the seasons. More with plenty food and cold weather, less with little food and hot weather. The best exercises are walking, riding, rowing, gardening, and not the athletic exercises which knock up the heart muscle.

Solid aliments must not be substituted by liquid aliments, be they tonic or reconstituent, beef extracts, milk, feculents, etc., because easily digested, for these latter do not sufficiently excite the buccal and intestinal mucouses. They may be useful to the Valetudinarian, to those whose digestive organ must be treated with caution, to the sick, yet here not for a long time, but they are harmful to the lad and the adult who needs strength, energy and muscles rather than an unnatural stoutness. Nevertheless, they perfectly suit old men who must try to keep up their equilibrium of health instead of looking for its increase. Liquids and vegetables do wonders with them. True old age begins at 63 years.

Thus, we must at any cost avoid to debilitate the organism, and nothing can substitute a mixed diet because, as the celebrated Dr. Maleschott says: "Flesh makes flesh." Man has absolute need of the products of Nature's three kingdoms, salt being to him as necessary as meat and vegetables.

The theoretical views extolled nowadays in dietetics cannot support the control of what Culpeper calls Dr. Experience who teaches that it does not suffice to ascertain that a substance contains azotated principles in order to be a substitute to meat. Indeed, in order to be able to establish a criterion between them, it is necessary that this substance be absorbed in such a quantity that no stomach can support. Still, meat diet is necessary, and animates, whereas lentils, beans, oats, soja, and cheese to excess, overload the stomach, and do not satisfy the spirit. This may be easily understood when one considers that the animal is a living pile whose blood is composed of the principles of the vegetables it browses, and that these vegetables through the animal organism are vitalized, i.e., dynamized. So that he who eats meat takes advantage of the principles of the plants vitalized through the animal body. That is the reason which led the celebrated Dr. Buchan to preconize in the cure of consumptives the milk and meat of animals browsing the herbs of an artificial pasture composed of herbs possessing therapeutical properties. Again, it is a flagrant mistake, except for some kitchen garden salads which yet are modified in their crudity by oil and vinegar or lemon or sauces, to praise uncooked vegetables or meat, because our organism needs cooked foods.

In fact, the fire, as a purifying and modifying agent of things, not only strikes off the noxious principles contained in raw substances but through the fragrancy it produces by their cooking it stimulates the gastric juices and anticipates the digestion. Thus, this latter takes place first through the nose, second through the palate, and third in the stomach and bowels.

Moreover, although foods ought to be well crushed in the mouth before their swallowing, it is not to say that they must be chewed until one becomes fatigued. This does more harm than good, because the stomach calls for working, and when the foods are reduced into fluid by mastication we deprive it of so doing, and prejudice it.

Thus I cannot too much extoll for anyone who is haunted by alimentary humbugs to take advantage of the following advice of Dr. Schofield: "Guided by these magic questions: Do you like it? Does it like you?" The pilgrim through life can thread his way through forests of food without encountering the giant of dyspepsia."

As to the hyper- and hypo-acidity of the gastric juices, they are only transitory and disappear as soon as the organ or organic system of which they are a reflex symptom is cured. They frequently depend on an abdominal plethora[1] and the orgasm of the vena-porta resulting from a default of the diaphragmatic breathing, and with women from a uterine trouble.

The milk diet in pyrexias is banished by the ancient physicians Hippocrates, Celsius, Cullen, Helvetius, and Piquer, and Hippocrates says: "Milk is contrary to those who suffer from violent headaches, fever, from meteorism of the hypochondria, from the throat, from bilious dejections and to those who lose blood from the fundament."

---

1 The sanguine plethora produces the leanness, and the serous plethora the obesity.

The Hygiene

Chapter XIV

Health and Beauty

Coming events cast their Shadows before.

Here are some directions for keeping healthy and fit and preserving yourself from the ravages of time.

Every year, from March 21 to May 21, take an amount equal in size to a pea, every three hours, of:

Natrum sulphuricum 2 X trituration. This keeps the bowels free and immune from acute diseases during the year.

If the summer is too hot and pushes to congestions:
    Gelsenium sempervirens
    Cactus grandiflorus

Add five drops in a glassful of water, a sip three or four times a day. And as preventive against sunstroke, put in the ears, first in one and then in the other, a plug of cotton soaked with arnicated water (1 tsp. arnica, 1 glass water).

Against the predisposition to take cold in the nose, rub the inner nostrils every night before going to bed with fluid extract of eucalyptus glubulus.

Wash the mouth every morning with 1 glass tepid water to

which is added 5 drops camphor water, and brush softly the teeth with sodium bicarbonate.

Once a month wash the hair with sunlight soap and half the quantity of the following filtered decoction:
    6 pinches powdered quillaja saponaria (soop tree bark)
    4 pounds water

Use the remaining half of the decoction to get off the soap. Rub afterward the scalp with an absorbent cotton soaked with camphorated ammonia fluid. The camphorated pomatum cures the itch of the scalp, if any.

Against the predisposition to costiveness, Jupiter collinsonia XI. Five drops in a spoonful of water, 4 times a day, and first thing in the morning, an enema with linseed water 2 pounds, aloes 3 grains, and when cold add: 1 spoonful of olive oil, beaten with the yolk of an egg.

Against anaemia, nervousness, neurasthenia, or sleeplessness:
Ferrum iodatum	2 X trit. 4 parts
Phosphorus	4 X id. 3 id.
Sulphur tinctura	1 part
Cuscuta europea	3 X id. 1 id.
Igniatia amara	3 X id. 2 parts
Avena sativa	id. 2 id.

Mix thoroughly, triturating half an hour. The size of a pea, 3 times a day. Friction morning and evening the neck, the spine, the loins with either *eau de cologne* or camphor water or salted water (1 teaspoonful for 2 pounds). Each day a walk of an hour, and once a week a chalybeate bath. Daily tepid baths promote sleep. With soups or apart, 3 or 4 spoonfuls of horse meat juice obtained through a digestor in hot-water bath, with a part of veal calf and some slices of carrots.

Against stomach troubles, take after meal a borage tea with 2 or 3 drops of orange flowers, water, and if difficult digestion or

Health and Beauty

stomacal pain: nux vomica 3 X, cinchona 3 X, sulphur 6 X. Add 5 drops in a spoonful of water before meals and on retiring. Rest of 20 minutes after meals.

Against neuralgia, rheumatism, etc.

Plantago major	3 X
Arctium loppa	3 X
Gelsemium	3 X
Veratrum viride	3 X
Colchicum	3 X
Viscum album	5 X

Combine and add 10 drops to a glass of water; take a spoonful every two or three hours.

For the complexion and the skin, wash the face before going to bed with soft tepid water, and apply with smooth muslin of the following preparation, letting it dry on:

Incense, powdered, 50 grams
Benzoin, powdered, 50 grams
Gum arabic, powdered, 50 grams
Sweet almonds, crusted, 80 grams
Cloves, crusted, 26 grams
Nutmeg, crusted, 26 grams
Pure rose water, 1 ounce 1/2
Alcohol 60°, 8 ounces

Filter and keep well corked. Iris versicolor, 6 X dilution, 10 drops, in a spoonful of water, three times a day.

For the eyes, a tepid eye bath, morning and evening, and if they are inflamed and congestioned, three times a day eye baths as warm as possible.

If weakened vision or threatened of cataract, use the following small battery:

Take an empty ounce bottle, and fill it full of white cotton batting saturated with a drachm of mustard oil. Cork tightly when not in use.

Hold the mouth of the bottle near the open eyes, first one and then the other, until the tears flow freely. Repeat three or four times a day. If there is a sense of over-stimulation, lessen the number of treatments.

This induces a renewed action of the nerves, muscles, and blood vessels, and a return of natural vigor to the parts. (Dr. Mary Ries Melendy)

During the period of change of life in both man and woman, this treatment in connection with outdoor life, Turkish or Russian baths concluding with a dash of cold water and simple cooling food will insure good vision in old age, without glasses.

Wear always a flannel coat or a tricot on the body.

As to the hygiene and therapeutics of the seasons:

Spring—eat less
   Remedies: aconit, 3 X; natrum sulf, 3 X

Summer—eat more salads and cooked vegetables with either butter or gravy or broth, and less meat.
   Remedies: glonoin 3 X; gelsemium 3 X; bryonia 3 X

Autumn—same as in summer, and moderate for fruits unless they are very ripe.
   Remedies: baptisia 3 X; cimicifuga 3 X; mercurius 5 X

Winter—safely satisfy your appetite and intelligently do provision of fuel for the year.
   Remedies: thus tox 5 X; ipeca 4 X; pulsatilla 4 X

Drink always abundantly during and after meals, either water with wine, or water with a few drops or old brandy, or Bass' or Alsopp's Pale Ale with water. Those who are lean must drink more during meals and less after meals, and those who are stout, nothing during meals, but after.

The wine must be natural and two or three years old. Graves, Moselle, and Rhenishwine suit those who do not urinate sufficiently, and Claret and Burgundy for everybody, if according to each temperament they are more or less diluted with water and taken only pure after meals, and no more than a wine glassful.

Use tepid baths. They are always and in any way profitable to health, and remember that balnea, vina, Venus, corrumpant corpora nostra, whether used in excess, and conservant cadem, balnea, vina, Venus, whether used sparingly.

Health and Beauty

Chapter XV

Periodicity

Nature never contradicts upon one plane what she asserts upon another plane. —Henry Clay Hodges, *Science and Key of Life*

The tendency of certain phenomena of living bodies to recur at stated times such as the budding of plants, the catamenia, the sleep, etc., marks this great law of Nature which governs all things and beings of the creation, and which depends upon the planetary periods.

I will expose some points practically useful in medicine.

The remedies that especially have a periodic action are agaricus, alumina, anacardium, antimonium crudum, argentum, arnica, arsenicum, asarum, baryta ear, cactus, calcarea carb, cantharis, capsicum, carbo veg, cedron, chinium sulf, cuprum, ignatia, ipeca, lycopodium, natrum muriat, nitri acidum, nux vom, phosphorus, plumbum, pulsatilla, rhododendron, rhus tox, sabadilla, sepia, silicea, spigelia, stannum, staphisagria, sulfur, thuya, valeriana, veratrom alb.

For a trouble appearing regularly at the same hour: aranea diad, cedron.

Every second day: alumina, calcarea carbo (evenings), phosborus, chamomilla, ipeca, natrum mur.

Every third or fourth day: aurom.

Every third day: eupatorium perf.

Every fourth day: arsenicum.

Every seventh day: arsenicum, aurum mur, catharis, cedron, crocus, eupatorium perf, phosphorus, sanguinaria, silicea, sulfur, tellurium.

Tenth day: kali phosphoricum.

Fourteenth day: arsenicum, kali phosphoricum, lachesis, niccolum.

Twenty-first day: aurum, magnesia carbonica.

Every two months: valeriana.

Every three months: kali bichromicum.

Every year: arsenicum, kali bichromicum, niccolum, rhus vernix, tarentula, thuya.

Every summer: lachesis.

Now I will terminate with a statement about the cycle of 36 years. The disastrous flood which took place in Paris in 1910 only had its similar in 1658 and 1802. Thus:

From 1658 to 1802, there are 144 years, i.e., 4 times 36.

From 1802 to 1910, there are 108 years, i.e., 3 times 36.

So the flood of 1910 is far from that of 1658 of 352 years, i.e., 7 times 36.

It is curious to observe the role played here by the cycle of 36 years, and the ternary, quaternary, and septenary, besides as the flood coincided with the return of Halley's Comet, let me cite these words of the engineer Bouquet de la Gyre pronounced 25 years ago:

> "It is with the waters' pathology as it is with that of the human liver. The waters may be affected by hypertrophy, cirrhosis; that is, the flood. And if through measures absolutely necessary, the period of hypertrophy of waters, which the comet will cause in 25 years, is not opposed, allow me, speaking as an astronomer, engineer, and hydrographer, to predict an overthrow of the French territory through the activity of waters produced by the astral influences.
>
> "This proves that all in Nature is subsidiary to the law of periodicity which rules the great clock of time—Saturn—of which we are unable to stand back or avert the progression.
>
> "During the great periods of calmness following hurricanes, man thinks he dominates the elements and forgets he is a straw whirling at the pleasure of the winds.
>
> "Only when it thunders is it that he remembers Jupiter's reign and perceives his powerlessness in the presence of the immutability of everlasting laws.

Bird's Eye Repertory

Drug's Affinities
(Analogous Remedies)

Aconit

With: antimonium crud, arnica, arsenicum, belladonna, bryonia, chamomilla, coffoea, dulcamara, gelsemium, hepar sulfuris, ipeca, laurocerasas, mercurius, nitri acidum, nux vomica, phosphorus, pulsatilla, sepia, sulfur, veratrum album, veratrum viride.

Remedies of less frequent use: aethusa, baptisia, cannabis indica, cimicifuga.

Arsenicum album

With: aconit, antimonium crud., arnica, baryta carb., bryonia, calcarea carb., carbo vegetabilis, chamomillia, digitalis, ferrum met., graphiles, hepares, ignatia, ipeca, lachesis, lycepedium, mercurius, natrum muriaticuram, nux vomica, petroleum, phosophorous, plumbum, sepia, silicea, staphisagria, sulfur, veratrum album.

Remedies of less frequent use: apis mellifica, baptisia, bro-mum, chininum sulfuricum, baptisia, kali sulfuricum, kali phosphoricum, kreosotum, iodium, muriatic acid, natrum sub-sulphurosum, ranunculus sceleratus, sambucus, scilla, secale, tabacum, tarentula cubensis.

Belladonna

With: aconit, ambra grisea, antimonium tart, bryonia, cale-area carb, cannabis sativa, chamomilla, china, coffoea, colchicum, colocynthis, conium, cuprum, digitalis, graphites, hepar s., hyosciamus, lachesis, mercurius, moschus, silicea, stramonium, sulfur, valeriana, veratrum viride.

Remedies of less frequent use: agaricus muscarius, cantharis, causticum, cicuta, cina, ferrum phosphoricum, helleborus, iodium, magnesia phosphorica, opium, phosphor acidum, plumbum, rheum, sassaparilla, senega, tarentula cubensis.

Bryonia alba

With: aconit, alumina, arnica, arsenicum, belladonna, calcarea carb, carbo vegetabilis, china, colocynthis, dulcamara, ipeca, kali carbonicum, lycopodium, mercurius, mezereum, phosphorus, pulsatilla, rhododendron, rhus tox, sepia, veratrum album.

Remedies of less frequent use: abies nigra, asclepias tuberosa, causticum, cimicifuga racemosa, clematis, ferrum phosphoricum, iodium, ledum, Millefolium, podophyllum, ranunculus bulbosus, scilla, senega.

Chamomilla

With: Aconit, alumina, antimonium crudum, arsenicum, belladonna, china, cocculus, coffoea, colocynthis, gelsemium, hepar s., igniatia, ipeca, lycopodium, nux vomica, petroleum, pulsatilla, rhus tox, stannum, sulfur, valeriana.

Remedies of less frequent use: boax, capsicum, cina, magnesia phosphorica, rheum.

Ipeca

With: alumina, antimonium crud, antimonium tartaricum, arnica, arsenicum, bryonia, calcarea carb, carbo veget, chamomilla, china, cocculus, cuprum, ferrum met, igniatia, laurocerasus, mercurius, nux vom, phosphorus, pulsatilla, veratrum alb, veratrum viride.

Remedies of less frequent use: drosera, euphorbia, hydrastis, leptandra, nitrum, opium, sulfur acidum.

Mercurius

With: aconit, antimonium crud, arnica, arsenicum, aurum fol, belladonna, bryonia, calcarea carb, carbo veget, china, coffoea, colchicum, cuprum, digitalis, dulcamara, hepars s, lachesis, laurocerasus, lycopodium, mezereum, nitri acid, nux vom, platina, pulsatilla, rhododendron, rhus tox, sepia, silicea, staphisagria, sulfur, thuya, valerina, veratrum album.

Remedies of less frequent use: apis mellifica, apium virus, argenium, asa faetida, calcarea fluorica, cicuta, clematis, euphrasis, ferrum phos, guaiacum, iodium, iris versicolor, kali bichromicum, opium, phosphor acid, phytolacco, podophyllum, rheum, sassaparilla, selenium, spigelia, zincum met.

Nux vomica

With: aconit, ambra grisea, arsenicum, asarum europoeum, aurum fol, baryta carb, belladona, bryonia, calcarea carb, carbo veg, chamomilla, china, cocculus, coffoea, colchicum, conium, cuprum, digitalis, dulcamara, graphites, igniatia, ipeca, kali carbonicum, lachesis, lycopodium, mercurius, moschus, natrum muriaticum, petroleum, phosphor, pulsatilla, rhus tox, selenium, sepia, stramonium, sulfur, valeriana.

Remedies of less frequent use: abies nigra, Aesculup hippocastanum, agaricus muscarius, aloes, ammonium muriaticum, caladium, capsicum, causticum, collinsonia, drosera, euphrassia, guaiacum, hydrastis, kreosotum, magnesia cabonica, millefolium, muriatic acidum, natrum sulfuricum, opium, plumbum, rheum.

Pulsatilla

With: aconit, alumina, ambra grisea, antimonium crudum, antimonium tartar, arnica, aurum fol, belladonna, bryonia, calcarea carb, cannabis sat, carbo vegetabilis, chamomilla, china, coffoea, colchicum, conium, cuprum, digitalis, dulcamara, ferrum met, graphites, igniatia, ipeca, kali carb, lachesis, lycopodium, mercurius, natrum carb, natrum mur, nitri acidum, nux vomica, petroleum, phosphorus, platina, rhus tox, rhododendron, sepia, silicea, stannum, sulfur, valeriana.

Remedies of less frequent use: agaricus musc, ammonium muriaticum, apia mellifica, calcarea phosphorica, caulohyllum, causticum, chelidonium, cimicifuga, cyclamen, euphrasia, hamamelis, hydrastis, kali chloruretum, kali sulfuricum, ledum, magnesia carb, manganum, millefolium, ranunculus bulbosus, rheum, sabadilla, sabina, senecio, spigelia, sulfur acid, verbascum.

Rhus tosicodendron

With: aconit, arnica, arsenicum, belladonna, bryonia, calcarea carb, chamomilla, coffoea, dulcamara, hepar s, lycopodium, mercurius, mezereum, nitri acidum, nux vomica, phosphorus, pulsatilla, rhododendron, sepia, silicea, sulfur, veratrum album.

Remedies of less frequent use: ammonium muriaticum, angustura, baptisia, causticum, cicuta, clematis, croton, hypericum, kali chloruretum, kali sulfuricum, ledum, phosphor acidum, ranunculus bulbosus, sambucus.

Sulfur

With: Aconit, ambra grisea, antimonium crudum, arsenicum, belladonna, calcarea carbonica, carbo veg, chamomilla, china, colchicum, coffoea, dulcamara, ferrum met, graphites, hepar s, lycopodium, mereurius, natrum mur, nitri acid, nux vomica, phosphorus, pulsatilla, rhus toxicodendron, sassaparilla, selenium, sepia, silicea, stannum, staphilagria, thuya, valeriana.

Remedies of less frequent use: aloes, apis, borax, causticum, chelidonium, kali chloruretum, kali sulfuricum, iodium, ledum, psorinum, ranunculus bulbosus, sassaparilla.

Veratrum album

With: aconit, alumina, antimonium tart, arnica, arsenicum, bryonia, calcarea carbonica, camphora, carbo vegetabilis, china, coffoea, colchicum, cuprum, digitalis, drosera, ferrum met, hyosciamus, ipeca, mercurius, phosphor, rhus tox, secale, sepia, stramonium, veratrum viride.

Remedies of less frequent use: camphora, cicuta, cina, drosera, iris versicolor, opium, phosphor acidum, spigelia, zineum.

Temperaments

Sanguine

Aconitum napellus, arnica, aurum fol., belladonna, bryonia, calcarea carb, chamomilla, china, cocculus, crocus, digitalis, ferrum met, gelsemium, graphites, hepar sulfur, hyoseiamus, kali carb, lycopodium, mercurius, natrum mur, nitri acid, nux vomica, phosphorus, pulsatilla, rhus tox, sepia, stramonium, sulfur, thuya, veratrum viride.

Bilious

Aconitum napellus, antimonium crudum, antimonium tartaricum, arsenicum alb, asarum europeum, bryonia, canabis sativa, chamomilla, china, cocculus, colocynthis, digitalis, igniatia, ipeca, lachesis, mercurius, mezereum, nux vomica, pulsatilla, secale, staphisagria, sulfur.

Nervous

Aconitum napellus, alumina, ammonium carb, arnica, arsenicum, baryta carb, belladonna, calcarea carb, carbo animalis, carbo vegetab, chamomilla, china, coffoea, conium mac, cuprum met, digitalis, dulcamara, ferrum met, graphites, hepar sulf, hyosciamus, igniatia, kali carb, laurocerasus, lycopodium, mercurius, moschus, natrium carb, natrum mur, nitri acid, nux moschala, nux vomica, petroleum, phosphorus, platina, pulsatilla, rhus tox, selenium, sepia, silicea, stannum, stramonium, sulfur, thuya, valeriana, viola odorata.

Lymphatic

Ammonium carb, arnica, arsenicum, belladonna, bryonia, calcarea carb, carbo veg, china, dulcamara, ferrum met, graphites, hepar sulf, kali carb, lyeopodium, mercurius, natrum mur, nitri acid, petroleum, phosphorous, rhus tox, sepia, silicea, sulfur, thuya, veratrum alb.

Seasons

Spring

Aconitum napellus, ambra grisea, antimonium tartaricum, aurum fol, belladonna, calcarea carb, carbo veg, dulcamara, gelsemium, lachesis, lycopodium, mercurius, natrum mur, pulsatilla, rhus tox, veratrum alb.

Summer

Antimonium crud, arsenicum, aurum fol, belladonna, bryonia, carbo veg, gelsemium, kali carb, lycopodium, natrum carb, nux vomica, pulsatilla, rhododendron, silicea.

Autumn

Aconit napellus, ammonium carb, antimonium tartaricum, asarum europoeum, aurum fol, bryonia, calcarea carb, china, colchicum, colocynthis, dulcamara, hepar s, igniatia, ipeca, lachesis, mercurius, nux vom, petroleum, rhododendron, rhus tox, silicea, stramonium, veratrum alb, vratrum viride.

Winter

Aconit nap, alumina, ammonium carb, arsenicum, aurum fol, belladonna, bryonia, camphora, calcarea carb, Carbo veg, chamomilla, cocculus, colchicum, dulcamara, hepar s, hyosciamus, ipeca, kali carb, mercurius, moschus, natrum mur, nitri acid, nux moschata, nux vomica, petroleum, phosphorus, pulsatilla, rhus tox, rhododendron, sepia, sulfur, veratrum alb.

Rulership of the Parts of the World1

Often in the treatment of acute and chronic ailments, the ruling sign of the country may be a useful appoint.

Aries
Denmark
England
Germany
Japan
Palestine
Syria
Florence
Marseilles
Naples
Padua
Saragossa
Verona

Taurus
Archipelago (Grecian)
Asia Minor
Caucasus
Cyprus

Persia
Poland
Russia (White)
Dublin
Leipzic
Mantua
Parma
Palmermo
Rhodes
Saint Louis

Gemini

Belgium
Egypt (Lower)
England (west of)
Flandres
Lombardy
Sardinia
Tripoli
United States
Wales
Cordova
London
Melbourne
Melz
Nurenberg
Plymouth
San Francisco
Versailles

Cancer

Africa (north and west)
Holland
Mauritius (east of)
Paraguay
Scotland

Zealand
Algiers
Amsterdam
Berne
Cadix
Constantinople
Genoa
Lubeck
Magdebourg
Manchester
Milan
New York
Stockholm
Tunis
Venice

Leo

Alpes
Apulia
Bohemia
Chaldea to Bassora
France
Italy
Roumani (norih of)
Sicily
Bath
Bombay
Bristol
Chicago
Damascus
Philadelphia
Portsmouth
Prague
Ravenna
Rome

Virgo

Assyria
Babylonia
Brazil
Crete
Croatia
Greece (part of)
Indies (West)
Kurdestan
Mesopotamia (Tigris to Euphrates)
Morea
Switzerland
Thessaly
Turkey
Virginia
Boston
Brindisi
Corinth
Heidelberg
Jerusalem
Los Angeles
Lyons
Norwich
Paris
Strasburg
Toulouse

Libra

Argentina
Austria
Caspian (borders of)
China
Egypt (upper)
Indo-China
Savoy

Tibet
Antwerp
Charleston
Copenhagen
Frankfort-on-Main
Fribourg
Johannesburg
Leeds
Lisbon
Nottingham
Placenza
Vienna

Scorpio
Algeria
Barbary
Bavaria
Cappadocia
Catalonia
Judea
Jutland
Morocco
Norway
Queensland
Syria (north)
Transvaal
Baltimore
Cincinnati
Dover
Franckfod-on-Oder
Fez
Halifax
Hull
Liverpool
Messina

Milwaukee
Newfoundland
Newcastle
New Orleans
Valentia
Washington

Sagittarius
Arabia
Australia
Dalmatia
Finistere
Hungary
Istria
Madagascar
Moravia
Provence
Slavonia
Spain
Tuscany
Avignon
Bradford
Budapest
Cologne
Narbonne
Nottingham
Sheffield
Stuttgart
Sunderland
Taranto
Toledo

Capricorn
Afghanistan
Albania
Bosnia

Bulgaria
Chorassan
Hesse
Greece
Macedonia
Mecklenburg
Mexico
Morea
Saxony (southwest)
Styria
Brandeburg
Brussels
Constanz
Fayence
Oxford
Port Said

Aquarius
Abyssinia
Arabia the Stony
Circassia
Poland
Prussia
Russia (Red)
Sweden
Wallachia
Westphalia
Bremen
Brighton
Hamburg
Salzburg
Trent

Pisces
Calabria
Galicia

Normandy
Nubia
Portugal
Sahara Desert
Alexandria
Bournemouth
Cowes
Lancaster
Ratisbon
Seville

Plants and Their Astral Rulers

Achillea millefolium: Venus
Aconitum lycoctonum: Saturn
Acorus calamus: Moon
Agave americana: Jupiter
Agrimonia eupatoria: Jupiter
Aloes socotrina: Mars
Althoea officinalis: Venus
Anethum foeniculum: Mercury
Anethum nobilis: Sun
Angelica archangelica: Sun
Apium graveolens: Mercury
Apium petroselinum: Mercury
Apocynum cannabinum: Saturn
Arctium lappa: Venus
Artemisia absinthium: Mars
Arum maculatum: Mars
Asparagus officinalis: Venus
Avena sativa: Mercury
Bellis perenis: Mars
Berberis vulgaris: Mars
Borrago officinalis: Jupiter
Ceanothus americanus: Saturn
Calendula officinalis: Sun

Capsicum annuum: Mars
Carduus marianus: Mars
Carum carvi: Mercury
Cichorum intibus: Jupiter
Cinnamomun (Laurus): Jupiter
Citrus lemonum: Sun
Crocus sativus: Sun
Cucarbita pepo: Moon
Daucus sylvestris: Mercury
Erythroea centaurium: Sun
Eupatorium aromatieum: Mars
Euphrasia officinalis: Venus
Fumaria officinalis: Venus
Hamamelis virginica: Mars
Hedera helix: Saturn
Helianthus annuus: Sun
Hibiscus esculentus: Venus
Hordeum hexasticon: Saturn
Humulus luppulus: Mars
Hypericum perforatum: Sun
Hyssopus officinale: Jupiter
Innia helenium: Mercury
Juglans regia: Sun
Juniperus sabina: Mars
Juniperus vulgaris: Sun
Lactuca sativa: Moon
Laurus nobilis: Sun
Lavandula spica: Mercury
Lenna minor: Moon
Lichen islandicus: Jupiter
Lilium candidum: Moon
Lonicera caprifolium: Moon
Lunaria annua: Moon
Lycopersicum esculentum: Jupiter
Malva sylvestris: Venus

Marrubium vulgare: Mercury
Melissa calaminta: Mercury
Mentha piperita: Sun
Mercurialis annua: Moon
Myrica cerifera: Mars
Nepeta glechoma: Venus
Nicotiana rustica: Mars
Nuphar luteo: Moon
Oleo europea: Sun
Origanum vulgare: Venus
Parietaria officinalis: Venus
Phaseolus vulgaris: Venus
Pimpinella anisum: Mercury
Plantago major: Venus
Polygonum hydropiper: Saturn
Polypodium vulgare: Saturn
Populus tremuloides: Saturn
Potentilla anserina: Venus
Potentilla tormentilla: Jupiter
Portulaca oleraccea: Moon
Prunus spinosa: Saturn
Pyrethrum parthenium: Sun
Quercus robur: Saturn
Ramunculus sceleratus: Mars
Rheum palmatum: Mars
Rosa gallica: Jupiter
Rosemarinus officinale: Sun
Rubia tinctorum: Mars
Sabatia angularis: Mars
Salvia officeinalis: Jupiter
Sambucus nigra: Venus
Sanicula officinorum: Venus
Saponaria officinalis: Venus
Saturea hortensis: Mercury
Scandix cerefolium: Jupiter

Sedum acre: Moon
Sedum telephium: Moon
Sempervivum tectorum: Jupiter
Senna officinalis: Mars
Solidago virga aurea: Venus
Sticta pulmonaria: Jupiter
Sisymbrium nasturtium: Moon
Symphitum officinale: Saturn
Taraxacum dens leonis: Jupiter
Urtica urens: Mars
Verbasum thapsus: Saturn
Viscum album: Sun
Vitis vinifera: Sun

www.ingramcontent.com/pod-product-compliance
Lightning Source LLC
Chambersburg PA
CBHW031434270326
41930CB00007B/706